Handbook of Orthoptic Pri...

Handbook of
Orthoptic Principles

G. T. Willoughby Cashell
Hon DSc Reading, MB BS Lond, FRCS Ed, FRCS Eng.
Emeritus Consultant Ophthalmic Surgeon,
Royal Berkshire Hospital, Reading.

Isobel M. Durran
DBOT
Formerly Orthoptist-in-charge, School of Orthoptics, Oxford Eye Hospital.

Assisted by
A. V. MacLellan
DBOT

Foreword by
T. Keith Lyle
CBE, MA, MD, MChir, FRCS, FRCP

FOURTH EDITION

CHURCHILL LIVINGSTONE
EDINBURGH LONDON MELBOURNE AND NEW YORK 1980

CHURCHILL LIVINGSTONE
Medical Division of Longman Group UK Limited

Distributed in the United States of America by Churchill
Livingstone Inc., 19 West 44th Street, New York, N.Y.
10036, and by associated companies, branches and
representatives throughout the world.

First Edition 1967
Second Edition 1971
Third Edition 1974
Fourth Edition 1980
 Reprinted 1988

ISBN 0 443 02200 3

British Library Cataloguing in Publication Data
Cashell, Geoffrey Thomas Willoughby
 Handbook of orthoptic principles. – 4th ed.
 1. Othoptics
 I. Title   II. Durran, Isobel Margaret
 III. MacLellan, Antoinette Vivien
 617.7'622   RE731   80–40527

Produced by Longman Singapore Publishers Pte Ltd
Printed in Singapore

Foreword

In all branches of medical work there is now much greater emphasis not only on early diagnosis and treatment of all disorders and diseases but also on measures which aim at their prevention.

Strabismus in chidren with its associated loss of normal binocular vision, and frequently with the loss of useful vision in one eye due to amblyopia, if early treatment is not undertaken, has in the past been much neglected largely because of an inadequate appreciation of the simple principles relating to its investigation and treatment. A book of modest size such as this which describes in simple terms the principles involved in the management of cases of strabismus with special emphasis on orthoptic investigation and treatment is most welcome and should be a useful introductory guide to the subject.

It gives me pleasure to write this brief foreword and to wish the authors every success in their undertaking.

1967

T. Keith Lyle

Preface to the Fourth Edition

In preparing this fourth edition the authors have carefully retained the original characteristics of the book – the chief of which are logical thought and economy of words.

The principal shift in emphasis since the appearance of the third edition has been prompted by a greater clinical awareness of the significance of the work of physiologists on visual development. This has contributed greatly to our understanding of the causes and effect of amblyopia and resulted in our reconsideration of its treatment. It seemed to the authors that these new attitudes to the influence on treatment of the stage of visual development reached by the young amblyope, warranted a rearrangement of subject matter: the question of visual acuity and amblyopia is now primarily dealt with in one specialised chapter. In addition the whole text has been carefully revised and updated, including the adoption of the new nomenclature published by the British Orthoptic Society in 1980 – although the old terminology remains indexed for reference purposes.

Once again the authors have enlisted the collaboration of Mrs A. V. MacLellan, DBOT, and they express their gratitude for her stimulating influence, with particular reference to her wide experience of the visual screening of the very young. They are also glad to acknowledge the constructive and helpful comments of Miss Alison Hood, DBOT. They are grateful to Clement Clarke Ltd. for supplying Plates IV, V, VII and VIII and to Mr Ian Smith, Senior Medical Photographer at the Glasgow Eye Infirmary, for Plates I, II, III and VI. Finally they wish to express with sincerity their thanks to the staff of Churchill Livingstone for their very real and personal interest in the progress of this book.

1980

G.T.W.C.
I.M.D.

Preface to the First Edition

The need for an introductory text, outlining the pattern of binocular disturbances and the principles of treatment, has become apparent to the authors during the recent rapid development in this field. This book is designed to present a natural sequence of thought which relates cause to effect, effect to prognosis and prognosis to management. This panoramic view of the subject was the basis of the teaching at the Oxford Eye Hospital both for orthoptic students and in the postgraduate lectures which the Orthoptist-in-charge was invited to deliver to a section of the ophthalmological staff.

This handbook is not intended in any way to be a detailed textbook on squint care (such publications are already well known) but it is hoped that it will be used as an introduction, laying the broad foundations on which may be built the more intricate detail already so admirably described elsewhere.

The book is written primarily for the benefit of ophthalmologists and so emphasis has been laid on those aspects of the subject which particularly concern them; there has, in fact, been a careful selection of the information to be omitted and only the most fleeting reference compatible with comprehension is made to the tehnicalities which are the orthoptists' responsibility. An attempt has also been made to anticipate the questions which the authors have met in their teaching experience at the Royal Berkshire Hospital and at the Oxford Eye Hospital.

The development of the book has reflected the teamship which must exist between the ophthalmologist and the orthoptist in the successful treatment of squint. While each of the two authors has been primarily responsible for that which refers to his or her own professional role, there has been a careful collaboration throughout. The final text, therefore, gives as integrated a picture as possible of that co-operation between surgeon and orthoptist which is the basis of the modern management of binocular disturbances.

The authors wish to express their very real gratitude to Miss Ailie Marshall DBOT for her invaluable contribution to the final revision and preparation of the text. Her collaboration created a stimulating partnership to which she gave her time and knowledge generously.

They acknowledge, too, their debt to Mr T. K. Lyle CBE, MD, FRCS for his interest and for the Foreword he has so kindly contributed, and to Mr John Durran, FRCS (Ed) who assisted in correcting the proofs and whose comments throughout the preparation of the book were a constant encouragement.

They owe thanks to Miss Peggy White, Mrs J. G. Skinner and Mrs A. M. Duncan, who typed the manuscript, and for illustrations to the Medical Illustration Department, Radcliffe Infirmary, Oxford (Plate I), Clement Clarke Ltd (Plates II-VII), and C. Davis Keeler, Ltd (Plate VIII).

Finally, they thank most sincerely the staff of E. & S. Livingstone Ltd for their helpfulness, care and patience in producing this book.

1967   G.T.W.C.
                                                                        I.M.D.

Contents

11. Principles for the management of squint

1

Binocular single vision

Binocular single vision is the co-ordinated use of the two eyes in order to produce a single mental impression. In its widest sense the term merely implies the simultaneous use of both eyes, each contributing to a common perception, but if the binocular single vision is to be considered normal, there must be bi-foveal fixation. It therefore depends on the satisfactory structural development of both eyes and is achieved only if their actions are linked by strong physiological bonds. At birth neither of these basic requirements is fully developed and thus refined binocular single vision is not attainable by the infant—but under normal circumstances it will become established during the first few years of life.

There are those who consider that binocular development is a maturing of innate binocular ability while others believe that it is entirely a learned function. To whichever school one belongs, it can certainly be said that the foundations for the development of binocular vision are laid before birth but are reinforced by time and usage.

In recent years there has been much research into binocular development in infancy in an attempt to establish the 'critical age' before which lies the 'sensitive period' when binocular vision can develop or, alternatively, be damaged very seriously by lack of normal visual experience. Evidence from research in several countries indicates that the impetus to the developing binocular system dies away by the age of 3 years and great emphasis is therefore being placed on visual screening of the very young.

ANATOMICAL DEVELOPMENT

There are several aspects of ocular development still to be completed after birth, the following being the most significant from the point of view of binocular vision.

1. The retina and fovea are not fully developed so that visual

perception is poor. This advances rapidly in infancy but may not be accurately demonstrated at 6/6 till approximately 5 years of age.
2. The globe is only 73 per cent of its adult size, resulting in a physiological infantile hypermetropia.
3. The ciliary muscle is not fully developed until 3 years of age.
4. The medial recti are structurally more advanced than the other extra-ocular muscles.

In spite of these imperfections, by the age of 5 or 6 weeks the rudimentary foundations of binocular single vision have become apparent.

PHYSIOLOGICAL DEVELOPMENT

The eyes are linked at birth by only one unconditioned reflex and the whole complex mechanism of their co-ordination rests on a series of psycho-optical reflexes, which are conditioned, gradually becoming as firmly established as unconditioned reflexes but capable, during the developmental 'sensitive' period, of being modified. They depend on time and usage for their development and in spite of increasing knowledge it is interesting to recall Chavasse's assertion that they are in a state of 'flux' from 6 months to 2 years, of 'diminishing flux' from 2 to 5 years and become 'fixed' by the age of 8 years. The binocular reflexes are as follows:

At birth
The postural reflex. Fixation of an object is maintained in spite of movement of the head and neck by means of this unconditioned reflex.

At 2 to 3 months
The fixation and refixation reflexes. These ensure that an object which excites interest is fixated by the fovea; the 'active' element of these reflexes is concerned with the abrupt fixation of a new object of interest and the 'passive' element ensures the pursuit of a moving target.
The vergence or disjunctive reflex. Disjugate movement of the eyes in order to maintain binocular fixation of an approaching object is controlled by this reflex.

At 2 to 3 years
The accommodation reflex. This develops as the visual acuity and

ciliary muscle power enable a clear image of objects closer than optical infinity to be formed.

The corrective fusion reflex. Tiny adjustments of the ocular position are constantly necessary to maintain binocular single vision, and these corrective movements enabling fusion are controlled by the corrective fusion reflex. In everyday life this reflex is essential in the control of heterophoria (see below).

The relationship between accommodation and convergence

The close link which must exist between accommodation and convergence is obvious since both are concerned with the viewing of objects closer than optical infinity. In generalised terms any stimulus to accommodate is accompanied by a stimulus to converge and these two actions are not induced separately. The convergence induced by a stimulus to accommodate is called accommodative convergence and the term *AC/A ratio* expresses the amount of accommodative convergence that is associated with one dioptre of accommodation; it would seem that in the individual this is a fixed relationship.

Relative convergence, which may be positive or negative, is that convergence which enables a person to maintain binocular single vision in the presence of a refractive error or heterophoria. It can be used in excess of accommodation (positive relative convergence) or inhibited in relation to accommodation (negative relative convergence).

HETEROPHORIA

Thus, by the gradual perfection of both the anatomical and physiological development, the co-ordination of the eyes in binocular single vision is made possible and a clear, single image is maintained for all positions in all directions of gaze. There are several definite advantages which result from the maintenance of binocular single vision (Fig. 1). These are (1) the field of vision is enlarged, (2) the blind spot of each eye is compensated for by the other, (3) the combined binocular visual acuity is slightly greater than the uniocular and (4) a highly accurate assessment of depth is possible in stereoscopic vision.

Binocular single vision is achieved by the strength of the binocular reflex development enabling constant fusion of the two monocular images and not by a fixed alignment of naturally parallel visual axes: indeed this condition (orthophoria) is comparatively rare. Far more commonly there is a latent tendency for the visual axes to deviate away from the parallelism required for binocular single vision, but this

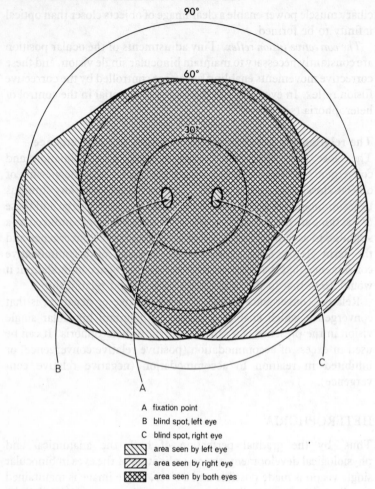

A fixation point
B blind spot, left eye
C blind spot, right eye
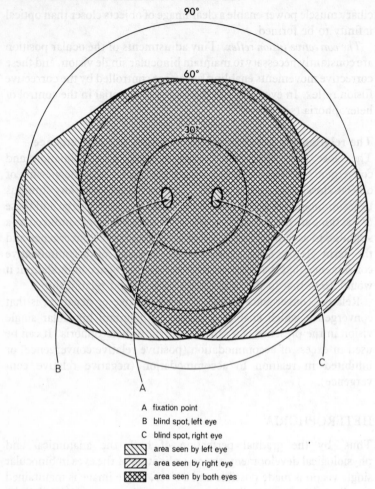 area seen by left eye
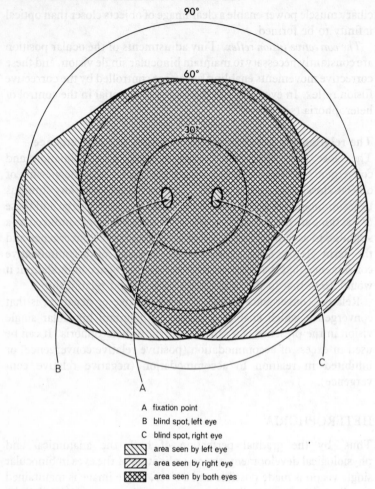 area seen by right eye
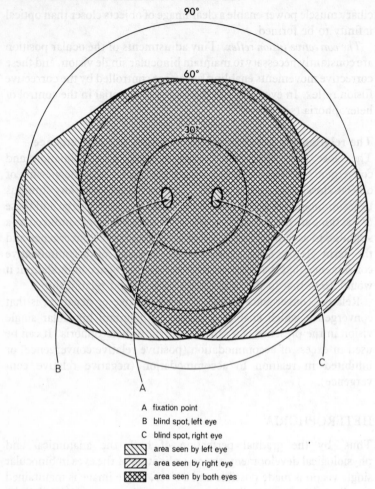 area seen by both eyes

Fig. 1 Representation of the field of vision

latent deviation, or heterophoria, is controlled by the strength of the fusion and is not permitted to manifest itself in the form of a squint. Very usually the eyes have a natural tendency either to converge (esophoria) or diverge (exophoria), occasionally there is a vertical element (hyper- or hypo-phoria) or, rarely, a tortional one (cyclophoria). However, this deviation in the vast majority remains latent and only reveals itself when bifoveal stimulation is prevented – for example, when performing the cover test (p. 16).

Heterophoria must be regarded as a physiological condition and most people remain completely symptom-free and quite unaware of the presence of a latent squint throughout their life.

RETINAL CORRESPONDENCE

If there is to be a fusion of the two monocular images there must be a physiological relationship between the two retinae; this is known as retinal correspondence, but in order clearly to understand this it is necessary first to consider projection (i.e. the interpretation of the direction of an object on the basis of the retinal elements stimulated) in uniocular vision.

In Figure 2

X is a fixation object stimulating the right fovea.

Y lies in the nasal field of vision and stimulates a temporal retinal element P.

Z lies in the temporal field of vision and stimulates a nasal retinal element Q.

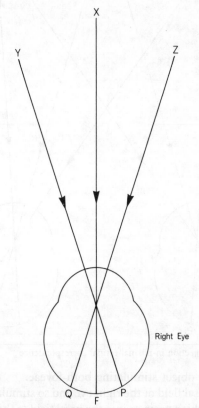

Fig. 2 Monocular projection

By normal projection, light stimulating nasal retinal elements is interpreted as having originated from the temporal field and vice versa. Similarly upper elements 'project' into the lower field and lower ones into the upper. Projection is to the same distance as that of the fixation object.

In normal binocular single vision projection is an elaboration of the same principle (Fig. 3), when a relationship between the two eyes, known as normal retinal correspondence, can be demonstrated.

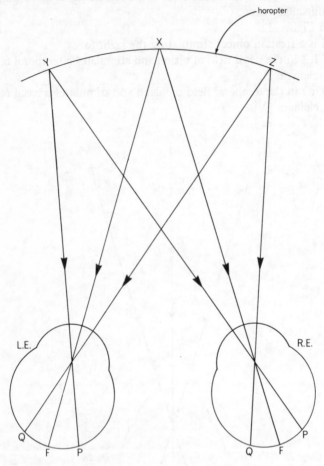

Fig. 3 Binocular projection in normal retinal correspondence

X is a fixation object stimulating both foveae.

Y lies in the nasal field of the right eye and so stimulates a temporal retinal element which projects into the nasal field to the same distance as the fixation object. It also lies in the temporal field of the left eye and so stimulates a nasal retinal element which projects into the temporal field to the same distance as the fixation object. The position of Y is thus determined by normal projection, and Z likewise.

Because Y has stimulated the points P on each retina and they have projected to the same position in space, they are said to be corresponding points. The horopter is the name given to the imaginary surface in space, all points of which stimulate corresponding retinal elements; it inevitably passes through the fixation object, which stimulates the foveae, and these are therefore corresponding points with 'straightahead' projection.

Physiological diplopia

Objects which do not lie on the horopter will not stimulate corresponding points, and, as non-corresponding points cannot

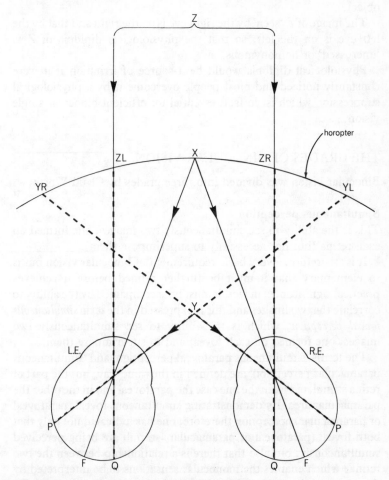

Fig. 4 Binocular projection with physiological diplopia

project to the same position in space, these objects are seen in diplopia which is physiological (Fig. 4).

X is a fixation object stimulating both foveae.

Y lies in front of the horopter and so stimulates temporal retinal elements (P) of both eyes, which project into their nasal fields to the same distance as the fixation object.

An image of Y is thus 'seen' by the right eye to the left of the fixation object and by the left eye to the right of the fixation object so that the images are said to be 'crossed'. This is heteronymous physiological diplopia.

Z is a distant object stimulating nasal retinal elements (Q) which project into the temporal fields to the same distance as the fixation object.

The image of Z 'seen' by the right eye is on the right and that by the left eye is on the left, so that the physiological diplopia of Z is 'uncrossed' or homonymous.

Physiological diplopia would be a source of irritation if it were constantly noticed and most people overcome it by a physiological suppression which is, in fact, essential for efficient binocular single vision.

THE GRADES OF BINOCULAR VISION

Binocular vision was divided into three grades by Claud Worth.

Simultaneous perception

This is the ability to see simultaneously two images, one formed on each retina (but not necessarily to superimpose them).

It is, therefore, a very basic requirement of binocular vision but is so elementary that it must be further refined before it achieves practical significance; in fact, it must be accompanied by the ability to correlate the two images and this is expressed in the term *simultaneous foveal perception*, which is the ability to see simultaneously two images, one formed on each fovea, and to superimpose them.

The terms 'simultaneous parafoveal perception' and 'simultaneous paramacular perception' are defined in the same way, but the part of retina stimulated is, in the one case the parafoveal and in the other the paramacular area. By demonstrating simultaneous foveal (parafoveal or paramacular) perception therefore, one has indicated not only that both foveal (parafoveal or paramacular) stimuli are being perceived simultaneously, but also that there is a relationship between the two retinae which enables the monocular sensations to be interpreted by the cortex as having originated from the same point in space. To exhibit the first grade of binocular vision, then, is to exhibit normal retinal correspondence.

Fusion

This is the ability to see two similar images, one formed on each retina, and to blend them as one.

There are two types of fusion: sensory (which simply expresses this power of blending) and motor, which is the ability to maintain sensory fusion through a range of vergences. It is extremely important to distinguish clinically between the very simple blending of sensory fusion and the true bonding of the image in motor fusion. The clinical method of diagnosis is described on page 86 but to make the difference plain consider a hypothetical situation in which there is bifoveal stimulation; whether there is simply sensory fusion or whether there is motor fusion these two monocular images will be blended (Fig. 5).

If a small base-out prism is now placed before one eye the stimulus

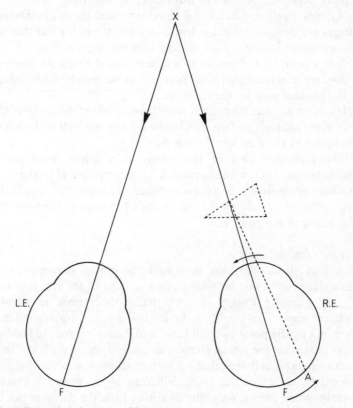

Fig. 5 Prismatic inducement of fusional movement

will be deviated from that fovea to a slightly temporal point A and the individual who lacks motor fusion will immediately experience diplopia. However, if motor fusion is present there will be a desire to maintain the single image and a corrective adducting movement will be made by the right eye to bring the fovea round to the necessary position to maintain the bonding of the two monocular images.

It follows that without fusion binocular single vision is impossible. Visual sensations are constantly moving and there is almost always a latent deviation to control; both these circumstances must be compensated for by corrective movements if bifoveal stimulation is to be maintained and diplopia avoided. The power instigating this co-ordinated and co-ordinating movement is the power of fusion.

Stereopsis

This is the ability to perceive two slightly dissimilar images, one formed on each retina, and to blend them as one with the perception of relative depth on the basis of this binocular disparity.

Whenever a three-dimensional object is viewed, the two monocular images are inevitably slightly dissimilar by virtue of the fact that the two eyes are viewing it from slightly different aspects (Fig. 6).

X is a point on the surface of a sphere stimulating both foveae.

A–C represents the part of the sphere's surface seen by the left eye.

B–D is that seen by the right eye.

It is apparent that the point X is well to the right of the centre of the area of the sphere's surface by the left eye and well to the left of the centre of the area seen by the right eye.

The binocular view of the sphere is a single fused image encompassing A–D, with the point X lying centrally and on the crest of what is recognised to be a curved surface. (This may very quickly be demonstrated by holding the cap of one's pen close to the nose, the clip acting as the point X.)

Panum's fusional areas

It follows, from what has been said concerning stereopsis, that binocular vision must be taking place in spite of the fact that two slightly differing images are stimulating the retinae in slightly different ways. This would not be feasible if retinal correspondence were on a rigidly point-to-point basis, and Panum's theory of fusional areas states that the retinal element in one eye corresponds not only with a single point in the other but with an elliptical area surrounding the exactly corresponding point. Whereas, by the theory of exactly corresponding points, only stimuli arising from the horopter can be fused, by using Panum's areas it becomes possible to fuse the slightly

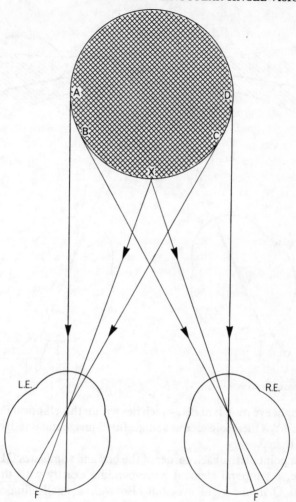

Fig. 6 Retinal stimulus by a curved surface

differing images seen by each eye when viewing a three-dimensional object extending into a narrow band of space in front of or behind the horopter. If an object penetrates beyond this band, retinal elements outside the limits of Panum's areas will be stimulated, and physiological diplopia will result (Fig. 7).

X is a fixation point on the side of a box and stimulates both foveae.

Y is a point on the front corner of the box and stimulates a point PL in the left eye. This is a nasal element having point-to-point correspondence with the temporal element P in the right eye, but also corresponding with a small elliptical area surrounding P. Stimulation

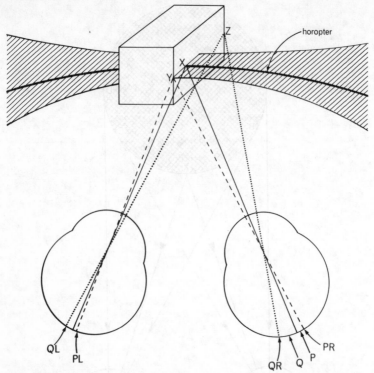

Fig. 7 Panum's areas

of the right eye by Y is at PR, which lies within this elliptical Panum's area, and Y is therefore seen as a single fused image and is judged to be nearer than X.

Z is a point on the back corner of the box and stimulates QL in the left eye, a temporal element corresponding exactly with the nasal element Q in the right eye, but also with a small elliptical area surrounding Q. Stimulation of the right eye by Z is at the point QR and the disparity between Q and QR is too great for QR to lie within the limits of Panum's area, so that two images of Z are projected to different points in space and Z is seen in physiological diplopia.

The shaded area in the diagram is the representation in space of the horizontal axis of Panum's area, i.e. any object lying within the shaded area will be fused and seen singly with the recognition of the third dimension. Panum's areas increase in depth towards the periphery and have a greater horizontal than vertical axis.

Fixation disparity. This is a condition occurring in binocular single vision in which the fixation object does not stimulate exactly corresponding points; the images, however, fall within Panum's areas so that the object is seen singly. This disparity can only be demonstrated under laboratory conditions.

Other theories

The mechanism of binocular vision is not yet proved and the principal opponent of Panum's theory of corresponding areas is the 'suppression theory'. According to this theory, retinal correspondence is completely rigid and one of a pair of corresponding points always suppresses the other; it is contended that depth perception is achieved by recognising the disparity between images seen in physiological diplopia. This suppression theory is of very early origin; Duke-Elder records a reference dated 1593, and it has only been challenged by the theory of corresponding areas during the past 100 years.

THE SIGNIFICANCE OF REFRACTIVE ERRORS

In the normal development of the binocular reflexes the state of the refraction is important as it may have a considerable bearing on any defects of muscle balance which may arise. The reason for this is twofold: firstly because, for proper binocular development—or, indeed, for monocular development—an image of maximum clarity must be presented to each eye; secondly because a refractive error will upset the normal balance which exists between the accommodation and the convergence.

It is significant that the ciliary muscle is not fully developed until the physiological infantile hypermetropia is reduced to manageable proportions. However, it will be appreciated that hypermetropia or myopia makes demands on relative convergence and the corrective fusion reflex if clear binocular single vision is to be maintained. Astigmatism or anisometropia, on the other hand, complicate even the achievement of a sharp retinal image and so can adversely influence not only the development of normal binocular single vision but also of the visual acuity. Refractive errors, therefore, require expert assessment and correction at a very early age, and 18 months is not too young.

2

The cover test

The art of prognosis and the skilful planning of treatment must always rest on an accurate diagnosis. In considering ocular balance a few cases have complete orthophoria, the vast majority have a heterophoria and a certain proportion will show a manifest squint. The cover test is a simple diagnostic test which reveals the presence of any ocular muscle imbalance—accurate assessment of the results of this test are, therefore, of prime importance in the management of disturbances of binocular vision.

The principle of the cover test is *dissociation*, an optical expedient widely used in orthoptic work, for both diagnostic and therapeutic purposes. This is a situation in which the stimulus to the two foveae is so altered that the normal ocular position, adopted in order to maintain binocular single vision, is temporarily suspended. It may be achieved by two methods; the first is by presenting each fovea with a separate stimulus with the aid of such devices as a mirror, a septum, a prism or complementary coloured filters. This type of dissociation is the more commonly used as it allows binocular vision to be investigated and treated during dissociation, while the alternative method—to dissociate actually by covering one eye—is to suspend binocular vision completely. However, it is this second (occlusion) method which is the form of dissociation used in the cover test.

Fixation positions
Fixation objects must not be so large that the patient's eyes may rove and should be clearly identified so that he knows exactly where he is expected to look; they must also be interesting so that the patient, if young, is tempted to sustain fixation. For children a picture is the most suitable, and if a question is asked which requires a reply ('look at that picture of a dwarf; is he smiling at you?') better concentration is achieved. Fixation objects are required in three positions so that any variations under differing circumstances may be noted.

The near position. The standard distance is 33 cm, which is regarded as the normal reading distance. Two types of fixation objects are best used in this position.

1. A detailed object such as a small picture or a series of letters size N6 or N8; these objects will induce accommodation and, since accommodation and convergence are so closely linked, it is essential to discover if the exertion of one leads to any disorder of the other. Useful fixation sticks printed with a detailed picture and a selection of letters in standard near test sizes (Plate III) are produced commercially.
2. A light; this does not induce accommodation and has the added advantage of producing corneal reflections. In very young patients a winking torch in the near position is frequently the only fixation object which will attract attention.

The distant position. This is at 6 metres or optical infinity. An obvious example would be the 6/60 letter or picture on the test type.

The far distant position. Any point beyond approximately 20 metres may be taken and is used in particular circumstances only (pp. 31 & 122). Again the object should be clearly defined and the patient should never simply be told to 'look out of the window'.

The occluder
The eye should be completely covered, or fusion of the peripheral field may prevent dissociation. In fact it is a good habit to use a small piece of card as this gives the examiner a crisp feeling of the exact moment of dissociation, when the deviation is to be noted.

Posture
In some cases an abnormal head posture is adopted for greater ocular comfort (p. 58) and in this event the diagnosis may quite well be incorrect if the cover test is only performed with the head held in the abnormal position. The test should first be carried out with the head held in this position and then repeated with it held straight for comparison. It is best to have completed the test with the abnormal posture before commenting on it because, once it has been remarked upon, patients find it difficult to return to the abnormal position consciously and a very important part of the investigation may be nullified.

Corneal reflections
These, resulting from fixing on a light, may be of help in very young patients who fix only fleetingly. The normal reflection is slightly nasal of the mid-pupil due to the slightly temporal position of the foveae,

but it is dangerous to draw too firm a conclusion from an abnormal corneal reflection alone, as this may be entirely due to an abnormally-placed fovea and not to any defect of binocular vision at all (p. 118).

METHOD

When examining a patient for the first time it is unwise to assume anything about the binocular or monocular fixation and so the cover test in every case should begin by investigation of these features. Only then may one safely proceed to examine either a heterophoria or a manifest squint.

Check for bi-foveal fixation

The patient is asked to look at a near fixation object; if binocular single vision is being maintained both foveae will now be directed towards this point. To check that this is so the examiner should cover the right eye, meanwhile closely watching the left eye; if the left fovea is directed towards the fixation object, the eye will not move while the patient maintains fixation. The occluder is now removed and the test repeated, covering the left eye and watching the right eye, when again there should be no movement if the fovea was already fixing. (This is the 'cover/uncover' test). If there is a movement noted in either eye, see Manifest Squint (p. 18).

Heterophoria

Having ascertained that bi-foveal fixation is being maintained, the examiner may now proceed to the cover test to reveal the presence of heterophoria. In this condition the visual axes are held in a parallel position by the power of fusion, but on dissociation the stimulus to maintain this position is removed; one eye will, therefore, slide away from the binocular position and take up what is known as the 'dissociated position'. This may be divergent, convergent, elevated or depressed. When binocular single vision is made possible once more the deviating eye will recover to restore bi-foveal fixation. The deviation is, in fact, a latent one.

To reveal this latent deviation by the cover test, dissociate by occluding the right eye and then moving the occluder directly to the left eye, repeating the process two or three times. This is the 'alternate cover' test and will demonstrate clearly the direction of any movement to assume fixation. Finally with the occluder once more obscuring the right eye, move the fixation object slowly from side to side as a final check that careful fixation is indeed being undertaken by the patient.

The latent deviation should now have occurred behind the occluder and, in order to observe it, the examiner must watch the right eye carefully as the occluder in front of it is removed. The eye will be seen to move back from the dissociated position of the heterophoria to restore binocular single vision.

If the eye moves inwards to recover it has evidently been divergent under the occluder and an exophoria is present. An outward movement to recover indicates a convergent position, or esophoria. A downward movement to recover indicates an elevated position, or hyperphoria. An upward movement to recover indicates a depressed position, or hypophoria.

Cyclophoria is a comparatively rare condition in which there is a wheel rotation of the covered eye. If '12 o'clock' has rotated towards the nose under cover it is known as incyclophoria, and when the cover is removed it will be seen to rotate outwards again. An outward rotation of the eye under cover is known as excyclophoria.

Figure 8 shows (a) the patient maintaining binocular single vision, (b) the right eye covered and diverging behind the occluder and (c) the restoration of binocular single vision by the uncovered right eye making an inward recovery movement.

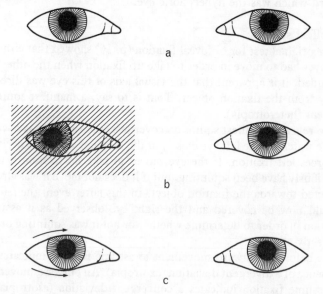

Fig. 8 Latent divergent squint

If the test is repeated by covering the left eye, the same response will be seen since heterophoria is not a defective position of one eye but a question of the natural position of the two eyes in relation to each other. Very occasionally inconcomitance may be seen (p. 57).

The test is repeated for near and distance with and without glasses and, in cases of exophoria, for far distance as well in order to exclude the possibility of intermittent divergent squint of the divergence excess type (p. 31).

Recording

The cover test record for a heterophoria should note the direction of the deviation as well as an assessment of whether it is slight, moderate or marked. Also, and this is important, an assessment is made of the rate of the recovery to regain binocular single vision. This last gives an indication of the ease with which the heterophoria is controlled

e.g. *with glasses*: moderate latent divergence with rapid recovery for near and distance; *without glasses*: marked latent divergence with slow recovery for near; moderate latent divergence with moderate recovery for distance.

If one eye is hypophoric the other will be relatively hyperphoric and, by convention, it is the hyperphoria which is recorded. In this case, unlike the horizontal deviations, it is obviously necessary to record which was the hyperphoric eye.

Manifest squint

If the original test for bi-foveal fixation (p. 16) showed that either of the eyes had to move in order to take up fixation when the other was occluded, it is apparent that the visual axis of this eye was directed away from the fixation object. That is to say, a manifest squint is present (heterotropia).

To reveal a manifest squint on cover test, the right eye is covered while watching the left eye closely at the moment when the occluder enforces left fixation. If the eye moves to take up fixation it must previously have been squinting, but if it does not move it was already directed towards the fixation object. In this latter event the left eye should now be covered and the right eye observed as it assumes fixation in order to determine whether or not it was squinting or was correctly aligned.

As before, an inward movement to assume fixation indicates the presence of a divergent deviation (exotropia). An outward movement to assume fixation indicates a convergent deviation (esotropia). A downward movement to assume fixation indicates an elevated deviation (hypertropia). An upward movement to assume fixation indicates a depressed deviation (hypotropia).

The test must be repeated for near and distance with and without glasses and also fixing either eye in turn. It should be remembered that if an accommodative squint is suspected particular attention must be paid to the near position, and in the event of divergence, the far distance cover test should be included in the investigation. If the cover test is carefully performed it should be possible to detect any of the variations outlined below.

A *unilateral* squint (Fig. 9) is one in which the squinting eye takes up fixation when the other eye is covered, but returns to the squinting position as soon as the cover is removed.

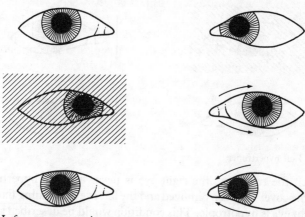

Fig. 9 Left convergent squint

An *alternating* squint (Fig. 10) is one in which the squinting eye takes up fixation when the other eye is covered, but it retains fixation even when the cover is removed, the previously fixing eye remaining in the deviated position.

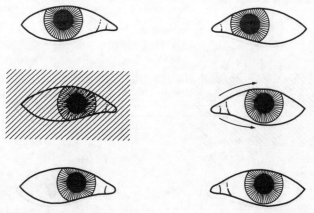

Fig. 10 Alternating convergent squint

The term 'alternating' is not applied to hypertropia in exactly the same way. Figure 11 shows a cover test on a case of left hypertropia, but the situation shown in Figure 12 cannot be described as alternating hypertropia because, although the deviation is alternating

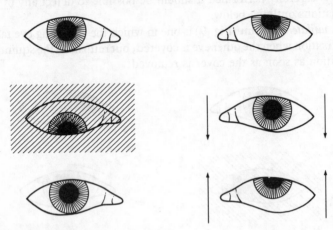

Fig. 11 Left hypertropia

between the two eyes, the right eye is never actually hypertropic. After the cover has been removed and the left eye is retaining fixation, the right eye is hypotropic. This condition would be described as 'left hypertropia with alternation'.

Alternating hypertropia is illustrated in Figure 13. When fixing with the right eye, before the cover test, the left eye is hypertropic and after the cover test the left eye has retained fixation and the right eye is hypertropic. This condition is normally associated with a horizontal

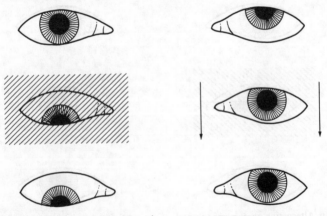

Fig. 12 Left hypertropia with alternation

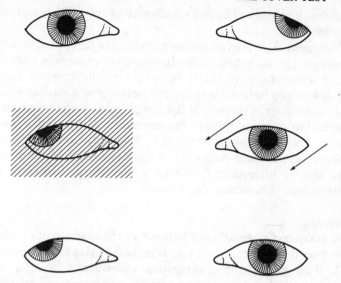

Fig. 13 Alternating divergent squint with alternating hypertropia

deviation, as illustrated. It should not be confused with alternating sursumduction (p. 31).

A *constant* squint is one which occurs at all times; it may be unilateral or alternating.

An *intermittent* squint is one which only occurs at particular times; it may be associated with a certain position (either near, distance or far distance) or it may only be apparent at certain hours—for example, when a child is tired.

An *accommodative* squint is one which is influenced by whether or not accommodation is taking place, or by the wearing of glasses.

A *concomitant* deviation is one of a consistent size, no matter which eye is fixing or to which direction the patient is looking. These squints are, therefore, non-paretic.

An *inconcomitant* deviation is one in which the size of the deviation varies in different positions of gaze, or depending on which eye is fixing. This is usually due to a muscle paresis.

A *microtropia* (p. 93) is a manifest squint of less than 5° in which a form of binocular single vision occurs. It may or may not be associated with an additional heterophoria so that on cover test there is a partial recovery only from the dissociated position, a small manifest deviation remaining.

The state of fixation. While carrying out the cover test note whether the patient is able, with either eye, to take up fixation rapidly and maintain it steadily. The full significance of this is discussed later (pp. 66 & 71).

Nystagmus. This is an oscillating movement of the eye and may also be detected on cover test. It may be latent, occurring only when one eye is covered, or manifest, being perpetually present. Latent nystagmus may be found with heterophoria or with a manifest squint and its aetiology is obscure. It is a complication in the treatment of squint, but does not prevent the maintenance of binocular single vision. Manifest ocular nystagmus is frequently associated with a defect of central vision (such a defect may be caused by albinism) or it may also be idiopathic; it will be a very severe barrier to the maintenance of binocular single vision.

Recording

The cover test record should indicate all the characteristics which have been detected during the test, as in the following three examples:

1. *With glasses*—slight alternating convergence for near and distance, increasing on accommodation; *without glasses*—moderate right convergence for near, reducing for distance.

2. *Near*—moderate latent divergence, rapid recovery; *distance*—moderate latent divergence, slow recovery; *far distance*—alternating manifest divergence with alternating hypertropia.

3. *Alternating convergence near and distance*, increasing when fixing left.

The cover test is the basis for the investigation of all cases of muscle imbalance, whether the deviation be latent or manifest, and its accurate performance should be a simple matter requiring only a moment of clinical time. However, the simplicity of the test can lead to a carelessness which all too easily results in a failure to make the correct diagnosis of the case.

3

Investigation of heterophoria

AETIOLOGY

It is almost inevitable that some degree of latent deviation from perfect orthophoria is present in at least some position of gaze in each individual, but, although this is true, the actual direction and degree of the latent deviation varies from case to case and is influenced by a variety of factors. Anatomical details, such as the inter-pupillary distance, and physiological factors, such as prolonged or neglected closework, may induce a tendency to latent deviation but, in addition, age will have its influence—esophoria being commoner in the young and exophoria in the old. Inconcomitant heterophoria (which may lead to an intermittent or even a constant squint) is often the result of organic, nervous or muscular disease, while the apparent triviality of a prolonged uniocular period can cause exophoria in an adult and induce a manifest squint in a child.

Refractive errors

The influence of these has already been referred to on page 13. In effect, one may say:

1. Esophoria is usually associated with
   a. bilateral superable hypermetropia, due to the accommodation it induces;
   b. bilateral congenital myopia, due to the proximity of the far point and the absence, therefore, of any inducement to relax convergence.
2. Exophoria may be found with
   a. bilateral acquired myopia, due to the reduction in the demand for accommodative effort;
   b. presbyopia, as the near point recedes and the bond between accommodation and convergence is weakened.
3. Cyclophoria may occasionally be caused by
   a. oblique astigmatism;
   b. incorrectly placed cylindrical correction.

DECOMPENSATION

It is only a small minority of the many persons with a heterophoria who experience any discomfort at all from the condition. The vast majority are completely symptom-free, or compensated, but for the few who are symptomatic, or decompensated, difficulties may be very real and severe.

Causes of decompensation

These are often not hard to trace and most of them stem from some form of general fatigue, associated often with either physical ill-health or mental anxiety. Thus the weary housewife overburdened by her work or the anxious father troubled by his taxes may suffer as severe a decompensation as is brought about by the more obvious factors, such as long hours of reading in a poor light. These fatiguing factors do not have their effect on the actual power of the individual muscles; the constant exertion of small corrective movements to maintain binocular poise taxes the fusional reserve rather than the ocular motor reserve. Increasing age may well result in a similar decompensation of a hitherto well controlled heterophoria.

Apart from decompensation due to fatigue, it may also be found as a result of what might be described as aggravating factors; for instance, an exophoric student who has spent the summer months in outdoor activities may find it difficult to resume intensive close work in the autumn. Also in this category the influence of both corrected and uncorrected refractive errors should be reviewed once more.

Consider the esophoric patient who gradually acquires myopia: while uncorrected the esophoria may have been well controlled but, once glasses are prescribed, the additional accommodation which they induce for close work will have the effect of increasing the tendency to esophoria. The symptoms are actually caused by glasses properly prescribed to correct the refractive error. Conversely, consider the exophoric patient who is slightly myopic and has a pair of glasses which he wears for driving and the theatre but which he imagines unnecessary for close work as he can see to read perfectly clearly. In fact this good visual acuity is achieved with little or no accommodative effort and therefore there is less stimulus to maintain convergence, so that the exophoric tendency is aggravated.

SYMPTOMS

A heterophoria which is decompensated is characterised by asthenopic symptoms, which occur after a period in which the eyes have had intensive use or at times of physical fatigue. It is not usual to suffer these symptoms early in the morning or after a holiday (although they may occur very quickly after returning to work). The symptoms fall into two categories: those due to either the maintenance or the surrender of binocular single vision.

1. Symptoms due to the maintenance of binocular single vision in spite of the difficulty in doing so.
    a. Headache (either frontal or occipital) or eye ache are the most common.
    b. Difficulty in changing focus from one distance to another is often noticed.
    c. Small inaccuracies in the judgment of distance may be a symptom.
    d. Photophobia is a very common symptom in exophoric patients who relieve it by closing one eye.
2. Symptoms due to the surrender of binocular single vision for fleeting periods in the face of the difficulty of its maintenance.
    a. Intermittent diplopia may be noticed, brought about by the temporary movement of one eye into the direction of the latent deviation. The patient is sometimes able to join the two images again but may not be able to do so.
    b. Blurring of print is usually caused by a relaxation of accommodation when binocular convergence to the page has failed. This may be associated with the diplopia mentioned above or, alternatively, the diplopia may not be noticed, due to suppression.
    c. Nausea or dizziness may be experienced with hyperphoria, as even fleeting diplopia is particularly troublesome if it is vertical in separation.

CLINICAL INVESTIGATION

After taking the case history with particular regard to the general health as well as to the nature of the symptoms, the clinical investigations will involve a variety of tests.

Visual acuity. This should be known before any other investigations are carried out, as it is an essential basis for the interpretation of the other tests. It should be recorded for near and distance vision with and without correction, if glasses are worn.

Refraction. If glasses are worn, information must be obtained as to how long this has been so, whether they are worn constantly or only for a particular purpose, and the date and strength of the present prescription should be ascertained. The refraction should then be checked.

Cover test (p. 16). The nature of the heterophoria is revealed by the cover test: the direction and degree of deviation (whether slight, moderate or marked) are of significance, but of very particular importance is the rate of the recovery to regain binocular single vision after the removal of the occluder.

Ocular movements. Movement into the nine cardinal positions of gaze should be investigated. (For further details see p. 96). This test is carried out binocularly and the movements are very likely to be full, but if there is any weakness of action further investigations should be carried out on the Hess screen (p. 100) by means of one of the several adaptations available. The Hess chart should be recorded so that an exact diagnosis can be made and so that a comparison is possible on a subsequent occasion to check for any alteration in the defect.

Convergence. This is measured on the R.A.F. near point rule (Plate I). The patient is asked to indicate when an approaching fixation line becomes double (subjective convergence having failed). The examiner should watch the eyes carefully to make an objective recording because if he has suppression the patient may not notice the diplopia when convergence fails.

Accommodation. Still using the R.A.F. near point rule, the patient reports the moment when an approaching block of print becomes too blurred to read (accommodation having failed). If the monocular accommodation is normal but the binocular poor, it is the convergence which is at fault, but if the monocular and binocular readings are both poor, the accommodation is defective. Accommodation should be checked binocularly and then monocularly, each test repeated three times to be sure that it does not fatigue.

Measurement. From the cover test an estimation has been made of whether the deviation is slight, moderate or marked, but it is now necessary to measure accurately the size of the deviation. To do this the eyes are dissociated so that there is no longer any reward for the maintenance of the binocular position; the dissociated position is then taken up and can be measured.

The prism cover test is a method of measuring the deviation by strictly comparable means in any position—near, distance, or far distance—by combining the cover test with the use of prisms, either separate ones in a trial frame or, far preferably, the prism bar. Prism bars are a series of graded prisms cast in two continuous bars—one with horizontal prisms and the other with vertical prisms. The prisms are used to correct the deviation revealed by the movement seen in the cover test. In this investigation it is best to cover either eye alternately with a continuous alternating movement of the occluder while the bar's position is adjusted until no further movement is seen. (For the principal of correcting a deviation by prisms see page 38.)

Prisms are used base-out to correct esophoria, base-in to correct exophoria, base up before a hypophoric eye and base down before a hyperphoric eye.

The Maddox wing (Plate II) is a near test and dissociates with the aid of two panels so that the right eye sees a red and a white arrow and the left eye sees two series of numbers. The patient looks through the eye-pieces at the white number 0 and, because the right eye will now have glided into the dissociated position, the arrow will stimulate either a nasal or a temporal retinal element, and will be projected accordingly. The horizontal deviation is measured by asking the patient which white number the white arrow indicates, and the vertical deviation by using the red arrow and the red numbers. Cyclophoria can also be measured by asking the patient when the moveable red arrow is lying parallel to the white numbers and taking a reading on the small side scale. Immediate dissociation is not always sufficient with the Maddox wing to reveal the maximum deviation and it is often wise to cover alternate eyes several times before taking a reading, as this tends to increase the dissociating effect.

The Maddox rod (usually in a handframe) is a distance test and dissociates by allowing fixation of a spot of light at 6 metres by one eye, but converting it into a streak of light by a series of red glass rods before the other eye. Also incorporated in the handframe is a rotating prism which will alter the relative position of the two images until they coincide. The horizontal deviation is measured by placing the rods horizontally so that a vertical streak of red light is formed; in the presence of a horizontal heterophoria the streak will appear to be to the side of the spot-light—homonymous in esophoria and heteronymous in exophoria. The prism, which was base down so that it had no horizontal displacing power, is now rotated until the streak passes through the light, and the scale reading is noted. The vertical deviation is measured by placing the rods vertically to form a horizontal red streak which can then be made to pass through the light by rotating the prism away from the base-out position, where it had no vertical displacing power. The Maddox rod should be used fixing either eye.

The Maddox rod (comprising simply the cylindrical rods) can also be used in conjunction with the tangent scale or in a trial frame with separate prisms, but these methods are not described as the

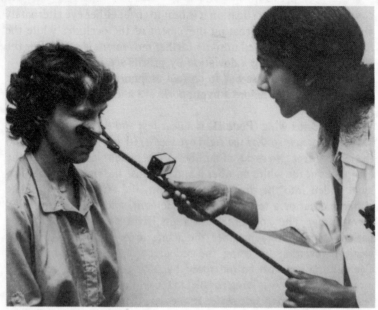

Plate I The R.A.F. near point rule

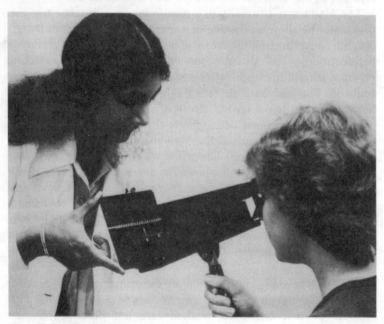

Plate II The Maddox wing

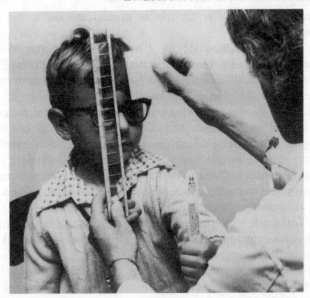

Plate III The prism cover test using a prism bar

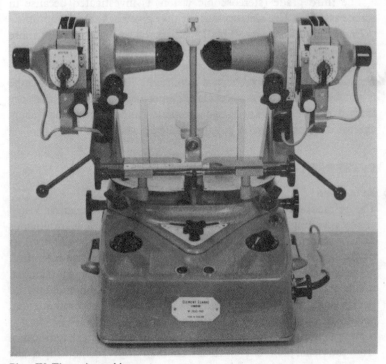

Plate IV The major amblyoscope

handframe instrument is the one in general use and is far more convenient.

The prism cover (Plate III) has a strong advantage over Maddox wing and rod tests since the dissociation tends to be more complete so that the maximum deviation which is being controlled is more readily revealed. This is particularly so if the deviation is at first overcorrected by using too strong a prism, which is then reduced.

The Major Amblyoscope (Plate IV). Investigation of a case of heterophoria on the major amblyoscope is important as it reveals the efficiency of the binocular function, and thus is an assessment of the reserves of control available to the patient. The technique of using this instrument will not be described here because it is within the province of the orthoptist's rather than the ophthalmologist's work.

The first grade (simultaneous foveal perception) is investigated in order to detect any suppression which may be becoming established as a result of the decompensation.

The second grade (fusion) is investigated in order to discover the strength of the fusional reserve—positive, inducing convergence, and negative, inducing divergence.

The third grade (stereoscopic vision) is investigated because in some cases defective stereopsis alone may give rise to the symptoms.

Prism bar fusion range. This is considered by some to be of more significance than the measurement of fusional reserve on the synoptophore. This is certainly true of esophoric patients when the negative fusional reserve is most important. The major amblyoscope is not best suited to its accurate measurement because of the very limited negative fusion range available, and maintaining fusion against increasing base-in prisms is more revealing.

INTERPRETATION OF RESULTS

Refraction

The refractive state is significant not only because defective visual acuity resulting from an uncorrected refractive error is an obvious disadvantage, but also because of the close relationship which exists between accommodation and convergence and thus, by inference, between hypermetropia or myopia and the heterophoria. The fact that uncorrected hypermetropia demands increased accommodation for near vision, while myopia reduces the need for accommodation, should be borne in mind when assessing the case.

Astigmatic and anisometropic errors are of greater significance from the visual point of view than from their direct relationship to any specific variety of heterophoria.

Direction and degree of the deviation

These are significant in that it is easier to control some types of heterophoria than others. Although no hard and fast rule can be laid down, there are certain suggested limits beyond which discomfort is likely to be caused by the effort to control. The cover test will have revealed the direction and an indication of the degree, which the Maddox wing, Maddox rod or prism cover test will measure.

Heterophoria has been subdivided into separate types, each with its own characteristic pattern of deviation:

Esophoria

Of the <u>convergence excess type</u>. The latent deviation is greater for near vision than for distance. In this case a deviation for near of over approximately 10^Δ may be the cause of symptoms.

Of the divergence weakness type. The latent deviation is greater for distance vision than for near. In this case control is even more difficult and a deviation for distance of 6^Δ–8^Δ may cause symptoms.

Exophoria

Of the convergence weakness type. The latent deviation is greater for near vision than for distance. A deviation for near of 15^Δ or even 20^Δ can be controlled without symptoms.

Of the divergence excess type. The latent deviation is greater for distance vision than for near; again it may be possible to control as much as 15^Δ without symptoms. *N.B.* If this type of exophoria is noted the cover test should always be repeated for far distance (i.e. fixing an object at least 20 metres away); a certain proportion of cases with a slight or moderate exophoria for near which increases for distance show a manifest divergent squint for far distance and fall into the category of intermittent divergent squint. Treatment for this condition follows a different course (p. 128) and therefore it is important that the diagnosis should not be mistaken.

Hyperphoria

This is the most difficult type of heterophoria to control because of the very limited range of the vertical fusional reserve, and a deviation exceeding 3^Δ is frequently very troublesome.

Alternating sursumduction

This condition, in which either eye elevates under cover, is not included in these remarks but is considered on page 153. In this type of case a vertical element of as much as 20^Δ or 30^Δ may be found without apparently causing symptoms and the condition should not be confused with the types of latent deviation discussed here.

Rate of the recovery

The speed with which binocular single vision is resumed during the cover test is of extreme importance, a rapid recovery denoting strong and easy control of the heterophoria, while a slow or lagging recovery indicates that difficulty is being experienced. In some cases of serious loss of control the patient may make no movement to correct the deviation after the cover test occluder has been removed until he has taken up a new fixation point, or blinked.

It is always important to consider together the degree of deviation and the rate of recovery; one patient with a 15^Δ exophoria of the convergence weakness type but a rapid recovery may be perfectly comfortable while another with only an 8^Δ exophoria and a lagging recovery may be very uncomfortable.

On the other hand, sheer size of deviation can be the cause of symptoms in spite of an apparently rapid recovery. A patient with a very marked exophoria, for example, 35^Δ, may show a remarkably rapid recovery in the clinic, but such a deviation will almost inevitably cause fatigue and symptoms by the end of the day.

Binocular function

Simultaneous foveal perception tests which reveal suppression suggest decompensation of the heterophoria since they indicate that, at times, the deviation is becoming manifest. This induces suppression to prevent diplopia. In extreme cases the suppression area is parafoveal, rather than foveal.

Fusional range, as demonstrated either on the major amblyoscope or with prisms, should be strong. The age of the patient must be taken into consideration here, but a positive range of 45° and a negative range of 5° should be achieved by a young adult.

Stereoscopic vision should be detailed and accurate. Poor stereopsis alone can be the cause of symptoms, particularly those concerning the judgment of position.

Ocular movements

If there is a limitation of any of the muscle actions (or if a nystagmoid movement is seen on extreme excursions) this should be carefully noted since movement should be full. If it is thought to be acquired and successive investigations suggest any deterioration, it could be that the decompensation of the heterophoria is the first sign of a neoplasm or disease. For this reason, any suggestion of inconcomitance, detected either in ocular movements or in the measurement of the deviation, should be treated with great respect, and further investigations immediately become indicated to determine the cause of the palsy.

Convergence and accommodation

Convergence should be well maintained to 6 cm in a young adult. Failure to do so may be an associated defect in a case of exophoria, but if it is an isolated failure it is not a case of decompensated heterophoria but one of convergence insufficiency. Defects of accommodation and convergence are a separate entity and will be considered in Chapter 5.

Symptoms

Specific types of defect are frequently associated with characteristic symptoms: esophoria of the convergence excess type and exophoria of the convergence weakness type are more likely to cause symptoms for near vision, while esophoria of the divergence weakness type and exophoria of the divergence excess type tend to cause symptoms for distance. It is also true that symptoms are more likely to occur after a period of intensive use of the eyes, and not after relaxation or sleep. However, this is not always the case, and a patient should not be dismissed simply because his symptoms do not entirely conform.

THE ROLE OF THE ORTHOPTIST

In the investigation of a case of heterophoria all the tests described, other than the refraction, may be delegated to a properly qualified orthoptist. She is also trained to assess the relative significance of the findings in order to judge whether or not the heterophoria is decompensated.

4

Management of Heterophoria

Correction of refractive error

Before considering the ordering of a spectacle correction, it is important to consider its effect on any latent deviation present.

It is usual for hypermetropia to be associated with esophoria and myopia with exophoria. In these cases correction of the refractive error will tend to decrease the heterophoria, and it is possible that glasses alone will relieve the symptoms. However, in considering the refractive error, special note should be taken of cases in which hypermetropia is associated with exophoria and myopia with esophoria, since glasses for these patients may well increase the size of the heterophoria and, while sharpening the visual acuity, may actually increase the symptoms. Thus when correcting a refractive error it would seem that the smallest possible correction compatible with good binocular visual acuity should be given to exophoric hypermetropes and esophoric myopes. It is clearly possible to make greater adjustments when dealing with hypermetropes. Conversely when prescribing for esophoric hypermetropes and exophoric myopes a full correction would be prescribed.

In all types of heterophoria a full astigmatic correction would be ordered. The type of latent deviation should, however, be taken into consideration when ordering a presbyopic correction. As the onset of presbyopia is frequently associated with a decompensating exophoria of the convergence weakness type, the lowest possible correction would be ordered in these cases.

It may be wise to have a full orthoptic examination carried out before prescribing glasses as it will give guidance as to whether a full or undercorrection should be ordered. It will also indicate whether a prismatic correction will have to be incorporated in glasses, and save having to represcribe after a short interval of time. The indications for the ordering of a prismatic correction are dealt with on page 38.

In cases of heterophoria it may be found that symptoms of decompensation are removed by the provision of lenses which correct the refractive error, and other forms of treatment may be unnecessary. The patient should wear glasses for a trial period of a month before further treatment is contemplated.

Selection for treatment

Before embarking on any further form of treatment it should be remembered that the mere presence of a latent deviation does not necessarily prove that the symptoms arise from it. Heterophoria is a normal condition unless decompensated and, in fact, perfect orthophoria is rare. Therefore, if there is any doubt after the initial investigation as to whether or not the symptoms of which the patient complains are in fact ocular, there are further simple measures which may be undertaken.

The occlusion test. The simplest, and probably the surest check: the patient is asked to wear an occluder totally covering one eye for a trial period of approximately a week. (It is best worn constantly, but if this is, for some reason, not feasible it should be worn as much as possible, and certainly at the times when symptoms are in the habit of occurring). Should the discomfort of which the patient has complained be caused by the effort of maintaining binocular single vision, this complete suspension of binocular activity will relieve all the symptoms. The patient may complain of difficulty in judging distance while wearing the occluder; this is quite normal, as stereoscopic vision is one of the functions which has been suspended.

Should the symptoms persist in spite of the occlusion some other cause for their occurrence must be sought and treatment of the heterophoria is contraindicated.

The prism test. Prisms are prescribed for temporary use which completely correct the latent deviation and thus remove any effort by the patient to control it. If glasses are worn, the most convenient form of prism for this purpose is the plastic adhesive Fresnel prism (p. 144), which is attached to the spectacle lens. Again, as in the occlusion test, persistence of the symptoms indicates that they are not due to the heterophoria.

Both these tests may result in an apparent increase in the size of the deviation. This is due to the prolonged relaxation of the controlling effort, unmasking the true size of the heterophoria. This further knowledge of the total extent of the latent deviation may well influence the decision to undertake treatment.

Exceptions

There are two occasions when treatment may be indicated in the absence of symptoms. If, in the course of some other investigation it is noted that a child has a latent deviation, there is a possibility of decompensation occurring later, and a course of orthoptic treatment may prevent that.

The question of treatment of persons whose heterophoria does not conform with the requirements for their career, e.g. the Armed Forces, is considered under Indications for Surgery (p. 37).

Orthoptic treatment

In cases of decompensated heterophoria orthoptic treatment is directed not towards the actual deviation itself, but to the comfortable control of that deviation by efficient binocular function. It is found that patients whose latent deviation is greater for near respond most satisfactorily to orthoptic treatment. Symptom-free control of large deviations for near can be taught, whereas even small deviations for distance may continue to give rise to difficulty. Clearly the size of the latent deviation must have some influence on the selection for orthoptic treatment, and large deviations in the presence of good fusional reserve will necessarily require surgery. However, it is impossible to put an actual figure on the size of the deviation that will or will not respond to orthoptic treatment, so, if appropriate, the patient should be warned before starting treatment that surgery may prove to be necessary. This is because in some cases symptoms may actually be aggravated by orthoptic treatment which alone does not prove adequate to restore comfortable binocular single vision.

The exercises the orthoptist will use in the clinic must be supplemented by conscientious homework practised by the patient if any success is to be hoped for, and therefore the patient must have sufficient intelligence and co-operation to understand, and carry out, what is required of him between attendances. His appointments should be weekly and an average of six visits is normal to gain symptom-free binocular single vision. The exercises fall into three main groups.

Anti-suppression. The foveal suppression, which has often developed during the period of decompensation, is a very real barrier to efficient binocular single vision and exercises to eradicate it on the major amblyoscope, using foveal sized slides, form a large part of the early stage of treatment.

Fusional training. This is of very obvious importance and is carried out by exercising the positive, negative or vertical ranges as appropriate on the major amblyoscope, with stereoscopes or with prisms.

Elasticity of accommodation and convergence. A variety of exercises has been devised to develop this essential element in the comfortable maintenance of binocular single vision. These are mainly dependent on the recognition of physiological diplopia so that the patient may fix an object in one position and accommodate to another. Exercises are given with stereogram cards without the aid of a stereoscope, or with lenses or prisms altering the amount of accommodation or convergence while the patient reads a near test type. Therapeutic instruments such as the Diploscope may also be used.

A detailed description of the selection of exercises or instruments and their technique is outside the province of this book as it is the responsibility of the orthoptist to manage the course of treatment for the patients referred to her. She will arrange for the patient to have regular visits to the department, where she will give a period of exercises lasting between 20 and 30 minutes and arrange the homework he is to do before the next attendance.

When the treatment is considered completed it is usual to allow three to six months to elapse before the orthoptist presents the patient to the ophthalmologist again for review and discharge. This is to allow a test period to be sure that the symptoms were not merely temporarily relieved by treatment.

Indications for surgery
A very small minority of cases of heterophoria will require surgery on their latent deviation; there are three groups of such patients.

Large deviations. This group comprises cases in which the size of the deviation is considered to be a major cause in the decompensation. Even a strong reserve of fusional power may be insufficient to achieve symptom-free control of a large deviation, but the symptoms will be relieved by surgery because that same fusional reserve is more able to control a smaller deviation. Pre-operative and post-operative orthoptic treatment may be combined with surgery in selected cases to improve binocular function.

Vertical deviations. Cases which are not considered suitable for prismatic correction, will require surgical treatment.

Service requirements. Particular ocular standards are laid down by certain bodies (for example, the Armed Forces) which have to be met by candidates for entry. If a patient has a heterophoria exceeding the degree quoted by the body concerned, there is no alternative to surgical treatment. Orthoptic treatment will merely increase the dynamic control of the static situation (and can, in doing so, mask the true size of the latent deviation) but it is the static defect with which the authority is concerned and this can only be adjusted by surgery. Orthoptic treatment is not indicated in these cases.

Surgical treatment

Surgical treatment of heterophoria will alter the size of the deviation but will have no direct effect on the binocular function. The aim of surgical treatment is to reduce the angle of latent deviation to a degree that will give the patient symptom-free control. It is possibly wise to under-correct the deviation so that the patient uses the same control mechanism as he did pre-operatively. For example if an exophoric patient who has always controlled his latent deviation by exerting convergence is rendered esophoric by surgery, he will find it very difficult suddenly to control his heterophoria by relaxing convergence.

In horizontal deviations results are more satisfactory if, as far as possible, operations are designed symmetrically between the two eyes. This may not always be possible when dealing with small deviations.

In vertical deviations the surgical principles are the same as are described on page 150 for paretic squint.

Post-operative treatment. A careful orthoptic examination must always be performed after surgical procedures on the muscles. Close collaboration is required between the surgeon and the orthoptist with regard to the continuation of orthoptic treatment, the wearing of the refractive correction or the modification of such correction.

Treatment with prisms

This is regarded as the least desirable means of overcoming symptomatic heterophoria because, whereas orthoptic treatment strengthens the binocular function and surgery reduces the deviation, prisms correct nothing; they simply deflect the path of the light entering the eye so that the fovea is stimulated by the fixation object in spite of the fact that the eye has deviated away from its parallel position.

In this way binocular single vision is maintained by optical aids while the deviation and the defective binocular function persist (Fig. 14).

In Figure 14(a) an exophoria is illustrated, the right eye having taken up a divergent position behind the cover, while the left eye maintains fixation of the distant object X.

In Figure 14(b) the exophoria has been corrected with a base-in prism so that the light from the object X stimulates the macula of the right eye in spite of its divergence. Thus both foveae are stimulated by X and binocular single vision is maintained.

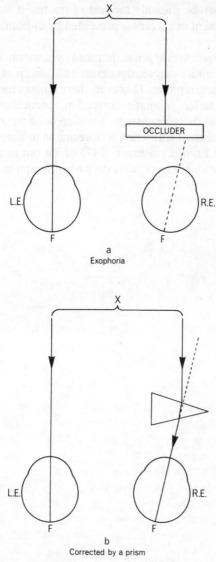

Fig. 14 (a) Exophoria. (b) Exophoria corrected by a prism

Indications for prisms

1. In small degrees of hyperphoria prisms can prove to be a very satisfactory method of treatment, as the size of the deviation does not warrant surgical intervention.

2. Prisms may be the only method of treatment available where orthoptic treatment or surgery is prevented by ill-health, age or some other factor.

Selection of the strength of prism. For many years authorities have felt it important to under-correct the deviation as much as possible, and yet eliminate the symptoms. However, there is now a feeling in certain circles that a fuller prismatic correction, particularly in vertical deviations, does not necessarily have an adverse effect. Before ordering a permanent correction it is desirable to have a trial period with clip-on or Fresnel prisms (p. 144) which can be adjusted until the exact correction which renders the patient symptom-free is found.

5

Defects of accommodation and the vergences

The ocular discomfort which can be caused by the decompensation of a heterophoria has already been described, but this is not the only reason why symptoms may occur during the maintenance of binocular single vision. The mechanisms of accommodation and convergence are also of prime importance, and defects in their action may give rise to difficulty.

Accommodative spasm
This is a condition in which the ciliary muscle is in a state of spasm, producing a pseudo-myopia. As well as the reduced visual acuity for distance, the patient complains of severe headaches and local discomfort or even, in marked cases, pain. In some cases diplopia may be present due to an excess of convergence. Accommodative spasm is not a common defect but is usually found in the presence of slight hypermetropia in young adults (or occasionally in early presbyopes) who are doing a great deal of sustained close work; it is frequently associated with neurotic tendencies.

On clinical investigation the distance visual acuity will be defective and the near point of accommodation may also be nearer to the eyes than expected. If routine refraction is carried out a surprisingly small concave lens (considering the visual reduction) will be found to correct the pseudo-myopia and restore apparent emmetropia. If this is inadvertently prescribed it will only aggravate the condition since it inevitably induces yet more accommodation. A refraction under a full cycloplegic is, therefore, essential, and the refractive error revealed, far from being myopic, will in most cases be slightly hypermetropic.

Treatment may be difficult and where possible the precipitating cause should be treated. Ocularly the patient should first be refracted under a cycloplegic, and a hypermetropic correction prescribed where relevant. In order to release the spasm and give a period of accommodative rest atropine 1 per cent is prescribed for a period of two to four weeks. In a few selected cases orthoptic treatment may help to stabilise the accommodation/convergence relationship after the spasm has been eliminated.

Accommodative fatigue

This is a condition in which there is a failure to maintain accommodation for close work. The patient complains of headaches and general ocular discomfort as well as an inability to 'focus on close work' and the condition is frequently associated with general ill-health or with poor working conditions such as inadequate lighting; head injuries and whiplash injuries can also result in defective accommodation.

On clinical investigation the near point may appear normal on first testing, but will recede on further measuring, and for this reason the near point of accommodation should always be tested three times in succession in all cases complaining of asthenopic symptoms. The clarity of the near test type will be improved by a small convex lens but will again blur after a few moments. Accommodative fatigue is frequently accompanied by a failure in convergence, although occasionally it may have quite the reverse effect and result in a tendency to overconverge, as a strong effort of accommodation is exerted; in this case the fatigue may occasionally develop into a spasm caused by the excessive effort to achieve a sharp retinal image.

Treatment again consists firstly of a careful refraction and the correction of any error found. The general health is often of significance and it, or any other precipitating factor, should also receive attention when, frequently, the symptoms will be relieved. However, they are likely to recur if the accommodation is not retrained under supervision and so a course of exercises should be given by the orthoptist who will govern the gradual re-introduction of accommodative effort and the establishment of a proper relationship between accommodation and convergence.

Variable accommodation

Unusual accommodative responses such as fluctuation or intermittent impairment may result from the use of certain drugs—including antidepressants.

Paralysis of accommodation

Loss of accommodation may be unilateral or bilateral and causes problems depending on the refractive state—more troublesome to the hypermetrope and of minor inconvenience to the emmetropic presbyope. It may be congenital but is usually acquired—either suddenly or gradually from nervous or traumatic causes or from drugs, infections or toxic conditions.

Treatment is first directed to the cause but miotics may help by stimulating the ciliary muscle as well as constricting the pupil. If the prognosis is poor, or closework essential during recovery, bifocals can be used with the correction calculated to encourage some attempt to exert accommodation.

Convergence insufficiency

In this condition there is a failure to achieve satisfactory convergence for the individual's requirements. The patient will complain of headaches and blurring for near vision, possibly throughout periods of close work but more commonly occurring after some time has been spent reading or sewing. Occasionally pathological diplopia will be noticed when the convergence fails but this is usually suppressed. Convergence insufficiency is a comparatively frequent disorder found in students or other persons whose working day demands long hours of close work, and also during the early stages of presbyopia. It may be precipitated by a period of ill-health, either mental or physical, and improvement of that condition may relieve symptoms, but is more likely to be due to unusually excessive demands on the convergence.

On clinical investigation there is, as a rule, a latent divergence for near vision but the distance cover test may not show any heterophoric response since it must be remembered that convergence insufficiency is not a variety of exophoria, but merely a dynamic failure of the power to converge, and may, therefore, be associated with exophoria, orthophoria or even esophoria as the static dissociated position. It should also be noted that there will be no limitation of action of the medial recti on testing conjugate side versions although the disjugate movement of convergence will be found to be below the standard expected for the age of the patient. The accommodation is very frequently slightly deficient too, since it will probably be relaxed when the convergence fails, giving rise to the symptoms of blurred vision for close work.

Treatment will open by correcting any refractive error, after which a course of orthoptic treatment is highly desirable. The exercises the orthoptist will give consist firstly of overcoming the suppression, so that the patient is aware of the pathological diplopia and thus recognises the surrender of binocular fixation, and then of improving the convergence. The accommodation usually recovers as the convergence is strengthened and the final stages of the treatment consist of developing that elasticity of the relationship between accommodation and convergence which is so essential for comfortable binocular single vision. The prognosis is good, but success depends on homework carried out conscientiously by the patient; often only four to six visits to the orthoptist are necessary, followed by a trial period without treatment before the patient is referred back to the ophthalmologist to consider discharge.

Convergence palsy
This condition presents a very similar clinical picture to convergence insufficiency but is usually sudden in onset. In the presence of normally acting medial recti it may be an early sign of a defect of the central nervous system.

Divergence insufficiency and palsy
Anomalies of divergence are quite rare, but deficiencies are usually due to prolonged excessive convergence or uncorrected myopia, while a palsy may be due to a structural lesion.

On clinical investigation there is esophoria for distance which will increase, and may become manifest, on progressively distant fixation but is always concomitant in varying directions of gaze. There is no limitation of abduction of either eye, an important distinguishing feature from a bilateral lateral rectus palsy (although cases due to a structural lesion may ultimately involve the sixth nerve nuclei). The thorough investigation of conjugate as well as disjugate movement is therefore most important, and any suspected divergence palsy will require full neurological investigation.

Treatment is not easy, orthoptic exercises not being helpful unless the condition is associated with excessive convergence. Prisms may be the only way of overcoming the diplopia for distance—prescribing the minimum strength which relieves the symptoms. Only if the condition is a palsy due to an organic neural lesion which is now static should surgery to the lateral recti be considered.

Defective dissociation of accommodation and convergence
The ability to dissociate accommodation and convergence and to exert them in unequal proportions is another important attribute of binocular function. Inability to do this may give rise to symptoms of strain and blurring. A course of orthoptic treatment aimed at improving positive and negative relative convergence, that is convergence in excess of accommodation and accommodation in excess of convergence, should relieve symptoms.

6

Cause and effect of squint

AETIOLOGY

Squint is a condition in which only one of the visual axes is directed towards the fixation object, the other deviating away from this point. Whether it be congenital or acquired, some influencing factor must be present which has prevented the normal development or the continued maintenance of binocular single vision. These factors were first drawn together by Chavasse in the seventh edition of Worth's *Squint* in 1939 when he discussed the causes of squint under the heading 'Obstacles in the Reflex Pathways'. His approach to the subject is largely followed to-day and no better classification for these factors could be found then the general terms 'sensory', 'motor' and 'central'.

Sensory factors

Much research is currently being carried out into the development of vision and this has lead to a greater appreciation of the damage perpetrated by any interruption to normal visual stimulus.

Dioptric factors

These may affect the formation of the retinal image, preventing the visual stimulation necessary to enable binocular vision to take place.

Refractive errors, if uncorrected, may be insuperable or superable. If insuperable, making the image blurred, fusion is difficult to maintain. This is particularly troublesome if the error is anisometropic so that the blurring of the two images is unequal. If the error is superable, the individual will make an accommodative effort to overcome the error, thus putting a possible strain on the relationship between accommodation and convergence (p. 3).

Opacities of the media, specially those affecting central vision, will have a serious affect on binocular function.

Retino-neural disturbances

Factors such as birth haemorrhage or other retinal defects will reduce the efficiency of the visual sensation and thus affect binocular control.

A monocular period

Bandaging or inflammation of one eye can have a particularly deterimental effect on a child (in whom the reflex development is not yet fixed). The same circumstances in adult life, or the use of monocular instruments for long periods are unlikely to cause more than decompensation of heterophoria.

Motor factors

These may affect the orbits, the extra-ocular muscles, the nerve pathway or the nerve nucleus.

Developmental anomalies

These are characterised by squints of congenital onset, although in some cases the mother may not be aware of the defect until the infant is about six months old because earlier non-alignment has been considered 'normal'. Such developmental anomalies affect:
the orbits as in

1. widely or narrowly spaced orbits,
2. facial asymmetry,
3. oxycephaly or telencephaly;

the muscles such as

1. incomplete differentiation,
2. abnormal insertions, distorting the action,
3. abnormal check ligaments, preventing full relaxation,
4. abnormal sheath structure,
5. fibrosis of the muscle tissue, reducing contraction and inhibiting relaxation,
6. aplasia or hypoplasia of a muscle;

the nerve pathway such as

1. anomalous connections,
2. aplasia or hypoplasia of a nerve;

the nerve nucleus, usually coupled with widespread anomalies resulting from cerebral defects.

Birth trauma

These are closely connected to developmental anomalies in that any resultant squint will be congenital. The trauma may affect:
the muscles

1. the lateral recti may be damaged in a forceps delivery,

2. haemorrhage within the orbit may result in fibrosis;
the nerve pathways or
the nerve nucleus by haemorrhage.

Disease or infection
Motor disturbances arising from such causes usually result in a squint of variable and fluctuating onset, possibly associated with local pain. Such diseases or infections may affect:
the muscles, either at the myoneural junction or at the muscle itself, as in
1. myasthenia gravis,
2. Graves' disease;
the nerve, as in
1. mastoiditis,
2. meningitis,
3. encephalitis,
4. disseminated sclerosis;
the nucleus, as in encephalitis.

Vascular disorders
These often result in deviations of fluctuating onset if haemorrhage or embolism was the cause, but tend to be progressive if caused by aneurysm or thrombosis. Those affecting:
the muscles are not common as an isolated cause unconnected with injury,
the nerve are most common,
the nucleus are often associated with more general disturbances.

Neoplasms
A gradual but progressive onset is the usual characteristic of deviations caused by neoplasms;
within the orbits they may cause a mechanical defect of movement by obstructing the rotation of the globe,
affecting the muscles by direct contact,
affecting the nerve, or
affecting the nucleus by pressure or direct involvement.

Trauma
This is a common cause of squint and is characterised by a deviation of sudden and dramatic onset, usually showing at least a partial spontaneous recovery as the immediate results of the injury are lessened. Trauma affecting:

the orbits is often associated with displacement of the globe (although this in itself need not cause a deviation from binocular fixation);

the muscles is not common as an isolated cause and is often linked with an orbital injury. It may occur without orbital injury to the lateral rectus, which is comparatively unprotected, or to the superior oblique at the trochlea;

the nerve may either result from direct injury—for example in fracture to the base of the skull—or from haemorrhage or septic infection. In the latter case the onset of the deviation is likely to be delayed;

the nucleus will very probably be accompanied by general defects besides the ocular deviation.

Central factors

Physical or mental illness

These are the most common central factors precipitating a squint, the effect of the illness being to undermine the general physical equilibrium and, in particular, the control which has hitherto been maintained of any latent deviation. This loss of control usually results first in decompensation of the heterophoria or an intermittent manifest deviation when particularly tired or disturbed. In an adult, it will only progress further than this if the pre-existing heterophoria was particularly large or difficult to control (for example, if a vertical element was present). In a child, however, periods of intermittent squinting tend to become gradually more frequent until a constant deviation may result. In many cases of squint occurring in childhood a central factor as well as a sensory one of the dioptric variety can be traced.

Hyperexcitability

This may be associated with a tendency to overconverge, again at first intermittently, at the times of excitement.

Hypoexcitability

This may be associated with a tendency to diverge; a proportion of children with an intermittent divergent squint of the divergence excess type are lethargic by nature.

Inability to learn

The fine and exact co-ordination of the eyes necessary to develop and maintain binocular single vision may never be achieved by some persons with insufficient ability to learn and a higher proportion of squints is found among children with a low IQ.

Ocular dominance

A factor which disturbs the natural ocular dominance can also result in a deviation.

THE EFFECT OF SQUINT

The presence of a manifest squint may have far-reaching effects not only on the binocular poise of the patient but also on the vision of the squinting eye, on the actions of the extra-ocular muscles and even on the bodily posture. The degree to which these resultant defects may progress is largely influenced by the age at which the deviation occurs and the period of time which elapses between onset and treatment. There is new evidence that the neuro-physiology of vision becomes permanently altered or impaired in cats and monkeys as the result of early barriers to binocular or monocular stimuli. Some 84 per cent of cells in the striate cortex have been demonstrated to be 'binocularly driven', i.e. they respond to stimuli from either eye and deprivation of corresponding retinal stimulus reduces their response. It seems likely therefore that man's visual system is similarly affected during the 'sensative period' of early childhood.

Sensory defects

Pathological diplopia

The immediate result of all deviations from binocular single vision is pathological diplopia. To understand this phenomenon, one must again consider the principles of normal projection (p. 5).

In Figure 15(a) an object X is being fixed bi-foveally and the point Z stimulates a nasal element of the right retina Q. This projects into the temporal field to locate the position of Z correctly.

In Figure 15(b) the object X is being fixed by the fovea of the left eye which projects straight ahead, but the right eye is convergent, the fovea being directed towards Y. Thus X stimulates the nasal element Q on the right retina and, as Q has a normal projectional value which locates objects as lying in the temporal field, a second image of X is seen to the right of the true object.

This is homonymous or uncrossed pathological diplopia since the image 'seen' by the right eye lies to the right of the image 'seen' by the left eye. This type of diplopia is characteristic of convergent squint.

In the presence of a manifest divergent squint the pathological diplopia is crossed or heteronymous; that is, the image 'seen' by the right eye is on the left of the image 'seen' by the left eye. This is illustrated in Figure 16 where the fixation object X stimulates the left

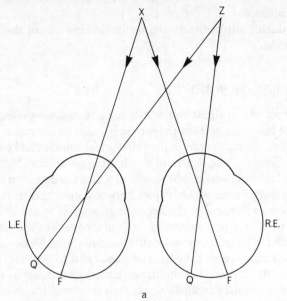

a

Fig. 15a Normal projection resulting in binocular single vision

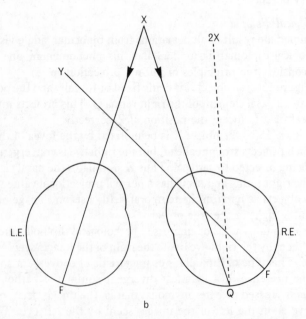

b

Fig. 15b Normal projection resulting in homonymous pathological diplopia

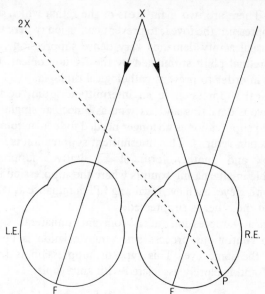

Fig. 16 Normal projection resulting in heteronymous pathological diplopia

fovea and is projected straight ahead, but stimulates the temporal retinal element P in the diverging right eye and is therefore projected into the nasal field.

In a case of hypotropia the false image will lie above the fixation object and in hypertropia it will lie below.

Confusion

This is not very frequently noticed by patients because of suppression (see below) but again, it is an inevitable projectional result of a manifest squint. It is the situation in which the object towards which the deviating fovea is directed is seen to be apparently superimposed on the fixation object. In Figure 15(b) it is shown that the right fovea is stimulated by the object Y and, as the fovea's normal projection is straight ahead, an image of Y will appear to be superimposed on to the object X, which stimulates the left fovea.

Suppression

The mental inhibition of visual stimuli, or suppression, may be physiological (p. 8) or due to pathological factors.

Pathological suppression occurs very rapidly indeed in young children, more slowly in those over approximately 6 years old, and possibly not at all in a patient whose squint develops after the age of 8 or 9 years. There are two main areas of the retina which are most quickly suppressed: the fovea, to prevent confusion (where the acute potential visual acuity demands very dense suppression), and the peripheral retinal point stimulated by the fixation object, which is suppressed in order to prevent pathological diplopia.

Pathological suppression in an intermittent squint occurs only when the eye is deviating and, as soon as binocular single vision is regained and suppression is no longer needed for ocular comfort, the normal function returns. This intermittent suppression is known as 'facultative', and another form of 'facultative' suppression is demonstrable in alternating squints where the suppression is always in the squinting eye, each eye regaining full dominance as it takes up fixation and the other is suppressed.

Pathological suppression in a constant unilateral squint is, however, a continuous process since the deviation is perpetually present in the same eye. This type of suppression is known as 'obligatory' and is closely associated with amblyopia.

Amblyopia

This is a condition of diminished visual form sense which is not demonstrably associated with any structural abnormality of the afferent visual pathways (including fovea and visual cortex). Much research into the physiology of vision and of visual development is currently in progress and it is postulated that amblyopia is caused by insufficient foveal stimulation rather than by active suppression of a disturbing diplopia. Certainly in contrast to suppression, which only occurs in binocular vision, amblyopia is found to be constantly present during monocular or binocular use of the amblyopic eye. This large and important subject is considered in detail in Chapter 7.

Acute vision develops as does a conditioned reflex and any interruption to this process results firstly in an arrest of development, and then a gradual degeneration towards extinction. Thus early deprivation of stimulus or the onset of a constant unilateral manifest squint will inevitably lead to the development of amblyopia, and this occurs more rapidly the younger the patient at the age of onset.

It should be noted that amblyopia is not so likely to occur in either intermittent or alternating squints, because there is not a constant neglect of either fovea in these conditions.

Fixation anomalies

Under normal circumstances it is the fovea which is used for fixation but in a certain proportion of cases of squint the fixation adopted by the squinting eye when it is forced to assume fixation is not central. In some cases this might be the cause of the squint, for example if the foveal structure had been damaged by birth haemorrhage or other pathological defect, but in many instances it would appear to be the effect. These are cases of untreated squint which have gone so far in the process of amblyopia that the sharp foveal visual acuity has been lost and is no longer superior to that at the periphery. It is among these cases that eccentric fixation is found.

Eccentric fixation. In this condition the amblyopic eye assumes fixation with a point other than the fovea. At first this eccentric point retains its normal projection but, as the condition becomes established, this peripheral point adopts the visual direction of the fovea. The visual acuity found in eccentric fixation is dependent on the position of the eccentric point concerned; if it is close to the fovea it may be physiologically capable of 6/12 vision, but the more peripheral the fixation point is, the lower is its visual acuity.

Binocular function

Fusion. This power degenerates in the squinting child because fusion, like a conditioned reflex, requires usage for its development until the age of 8 years, and if a squint prevents proper stimulus before that age this growth of fusion will be interrupted. At first its power is potentially available in spite of the deviation so that if the two foveae are once again stimulated by the same object (for example, if the squint is corrected, or with an amblyoscope, or prisms) fusion of the two retinal images is resumed. This potential power, however, degenerates rapidly in a young child until finally the ability may be entirely lost.

In cases of squint with onset during or after adolescence, loss of fusion is unlikely, since it was firmly established before the onset of the squint. The exceptions to this generalisation are cases of squint following traumatic cataract, who show severe loss of fusion within six months of the formation of the cataract, and cases of squint due to an injury which resulted in concussion, who may show immediate loss of fusion power.

Retinal correspondence. As was explained in Chapter I, fusion power is based on the normal correspondence which exists between the retinal elements in the two eyes, and, in the same way as fusion may degenerate through lack of proper stimulation, so may this normal retinal correspondence. There will be a period in which there is still a completely normal potential correspondence between the two retinae although fusion itself is already lost but, without fusion, this retinal correspondence is valueless to the individual although it is, of course, the essential foundation for the development of fusion.

Lack of retinal correspondence. When stimulation of the two foveae no longer results in projection to the same point in space but the perception of one of the images results in total suppression of the other, the patient is said to lack retinal correspondence. Rapid degeneration of binocular function to this level is, unfortunately, frequently seen in cases of squint of early onset unless adequate steps to prevent it are taken. When there is lack of retinal correspondence the most elementary requirement for binocular single vision is lost, for without retinal correspondence there can be no true fusion.

Abnormal retinal correspondence. This is a binocular condition in which the fovea of the fixing eye has a common visual direction with an area other than the fovea (sometimes called the pseudo-fovea) of the deviating eye. This condition occurs whichever eye is fixing and involves a change in the visual direction of all retinal points in the deviating eye. There are several theories explaining the development of abnormal retinal correspondence, but one which is currently held in favour is the theory put forward by Travers.

In the case illustrated in Figure 17 the object X stimulates the left fovea (FL) and the nasal element Q in the right eye, which are

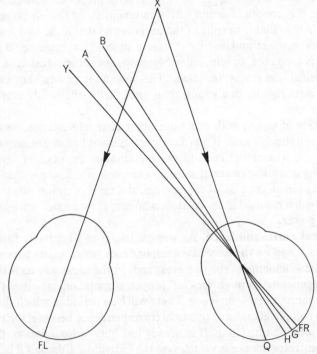

Fig. 17 Travers' theory

non-corresponding points. Q is therefore suppressed in order to prevent diplopia and the right fovea (FR) is also suppressed to avoid confusion.

Since the use of the two foveae simultaneously has resulted in confusion, an attempt is made to establish a correspondence between FL and a point G slightly nasal to FR; however G is stimulated by the object A and therefore confusion again results so that G is suppressed. An attempt is now made to correspond H with FL—again resulting in confusion between B and X. Gradually the suppression area from FR grows as successively nasal elements are used in an abnormal correspondence with FL until finally the point Q is reached. Now there is no confusion (since both Q and FL are stimulated by the object X) and a correspondence between these two points is established which results in an anomalous form of binocular vision. It is crude compared with that found in normal binocular single vision because it is a correspondence between a highly developed point on one retina (the fovea) and a peripheral point on the other, with comparatively poor visual acuity; thus the fusion and stereopsis resulting from this correspondence must necessarily be inferior; the more peripheral the non-corresponding point used, the more inferior the anomalous binocular function.

Harmonious abnormal retinal correspondence is said to exist when the point Q has been reached and the reorientation of the correspondence is complete.

Unharmonious abnormal retinal correspondence is present during the time of development while points lying between FR and Q 'correspond' with FL. The view is now being expressed that unharmonious abnormal retinal correspondence does not exist in free space but is only induced by certain examination methods.

Abnormal retinal correspondence is normally found in a unilateral convergent squint of early onset for whom diagnosis and treatment were not quickly enough made available; usually the angle of deviation is less than 20°. It may also be found in small residual deviations of under 7° where early surgery has been performed without subsequent total recovery to true binocular single vision (and some cases of microtropia may fall within this category). These cases are best left without further treatment.

A note might be of value here to emphasise the essential difference between two conditions which are commonly confused: eccentric fixation and abnormal retinal correspondence.

Eccentric fixation is a perversion of purely monocular activity in which a peripheral retinal element rather than the fovea is used for fixation. Moreover, the projectional value of this element has become re-orientated so that it has adopted the straight-ahead projection characteristic of the fovea.

Abnormal retinal correspondence is, in contrast, a purely binocular condition in which there has developed a correspondence between the fovea of one eye and a peripheral element in the other. In a simple case foveal fixation persists and the retinal elements have retained their original projectional value under purely monocular conditions, the perversion being one of binocular correspondence only. However, in some instances patients with abnormal retinal correspondence may also have eccentric fixation, but it is seldom found that the anomalous point used in binocular fixation is the same as the eccentric point used in monocular fixation.

Muscular defects

Non-paretic squints

These have occurred without any causal motor defect; they are very numerous and many cases show full movement of either eye in all directions of gaze. However, in longstanding cases some secondary defect of muscle action may reveal itself.

Excessive action of a habitually used muscle is common: in a case of right convergent squint, the right eye may show elevation on laevoversion due to the natural slight advantage which the inferior oblique muscle holds over the superior oblique muscle in that position.

Defective action of a habitually disused muscle may equally well occur and a common example is seen in the habitual disuse of the lateral recti in cases of alternating squint. (These patients tend to use the tripartite field of fixation: the convergent right eye for the left field, the convergent left eye for the right field and either eye for the central field).

Paretic squints

This group of squints (which are caused by a disturbance of the motor control of the ocular posture) also show changes in the muscular balance with the passage of time. These changes are the gradual effect of the phsyiological laws defined by Hering and Sherrington. Hering's law of equal innervation states that an impulse to one muscle to contract is accompanied by an identical impulse to the contralateral synergist to contract; Sherrington's law of reciprocal innervation states that any impulse to one muscle to contract is accompanied by a stimulus to its ipsilateral antagonist to relax.

Inconcomitance. Variation in the size of a deviation depending on which eye is fixing or on the direction of gaze is known as inconcomitance and is the characteristic of recently acquired paretic squints. Take, for example, a case of right lateral rectus palsy; when looking straight ahead and fixing with the left eye, the right eye will be convergent by a certain amount due to the paresis of the lateral rectus.

To illustrate the variation in the size of the squint which occurs with alteration of the fixing eye, consider the situation if fixation is now attempted by the right eye. A greater stimulation than normal will be required to obtain sufficient contracture of the right lateral rectus to achieve right fixation and, by Hering's law, this exaggerated stimulus will also reach the contralateral synergist (the left medial rectus) and will cause an exaggerated convergence of the left eye.

To illustrate the variation which occurs depending on the direction of gaze, consider the situation if the unaffected left eye retains constant fixation and if laevo-version is now attempted. The left eye will move normally, and the right eye will require contraction of the unaffected medial rectus accompanied by relaxation of the lateral rectus. As the lateral rectus is already paretic this direction of gaze causes no difficulty and the angle of squint is reduced, and may even be eliminated so that binocular single vision is maintained. Conversely, if dextro-version is attempted the left eye will again move normally but the right eye is now required to abduct, involving contraction of the paretic lateral rectus. As the stimulus to the right lateral rectus is governed by that to the medial rectus of the fixing left eye, the contraction of the affected muscle is very inadequate and the size of the squint is thus greatly increased.

In summary, therefore, it may be said that the angle of deviation is greatest when looking into the direction of action of the affected muscle, and when fixing with the affected eye.

Concomitance. In paretic squint concomitance can only be relative since there will always be a variation in the size of the deviation in different directions of gaze. However, in these cases the development of relative concomitance is an indication that the defect is of longstanding duration, for it is only by the passage of time that, gradually, this concomitance occurs due to the muscle sequelae. The sequelae are:

1. Excessive action of the contralateral synergist (by Hering's Law).
2. Contracture of the ipsolateral antagonist (by virtue of the fact that its opposition from the affected muscle is now reduced).
3. Defective action of the contralateral antagonist (due to the excessive overaction of the contralateral synergist enforcing its greater relaxation by Sherrington's Law).

To relate these sequelae to the case described in the consideration of inconcomitance, that of a right lateral rectus palsy, there would be:

1. Excessive action of the left medial rectus,
2. Contracture of the right medial rectus,
3. Defective action of the left lateral rectus.

Finally to relate the sequelae to a palsy of a vertically acting muscle, take, for example, a case of right superior rectus palsy. There will be:

1. Excessive action of the left inferior oblique,
2. Contracture of the right inferior rectus,
3. Defective action of the left superior oblique.

The development of concomitance can reach the stage when it is no longer easy to determine whether the truly paretic muscle or its contralateral antagonist was primarily affected. Indeed many congenital squints may have been paretic in origin due to neonatal accident but are concomitant by the time accurate assessment can be made perhaps two years later.

Thyroid dysfunction
The ocular muscle imbalance produced in thyroid dysfunction presents a clinical picture similar to some acquired paretic squints and it is therefore important to distinguish between them. Degenerative changes take place in the muscles leading to fibrosis and mechanical restriction. The muscle most commonly affected is the inferior rectus (preventing elevation of the globe) but the medial rectus or inferior oblique may be involved. There is usually exophthalmos and lid retraction together with typical asymmetrical limitations of upward gaze and diplopia. The patients commonly complain of 'stiff eyes', especially on waking, and pain when looking upward.

Postural defects
It has already been pointed out in the section on inconcomitance that a paretic squint is likely to vary considerably in size depending on which eye is fixing and into which direction the patient is looking. This fact may be used by the patient who limits the variation either by preventing the movement of his eyes into the most troublesome position, so that he can achieve binocular single vision, or by persistently looking into the direction where the deviation is greatest so that the diplopia is separated and becomes less irritating. However, it is not very feasible to hold the eye in, for example, perpetual dextro-version and so a compensatory mechanism is adopted in the form of an abnormal head posture.

Abnormal head postures are a means of enabling the eyes to be held in other than the primary position while yet maintaining a field of vision which lies straight ahead. For example, if the face is turned to the left while a central fixation object is viewed, the eyes will assume a position of dextro-version.

Horizontal palsies. These may be accompanied by a simple face turn of this nature; the turn to the left mentioned above could enable binocular single vision to be maintained in a case of mild palsy of the left lateral rectus, as dextro-version will be the direction in which the paresis will cause least difficulty. But it could alternatively be adopted in a case of right lateral rectus palsy which was too marked to enable binocular single vision to be achieved in any position; in this case the abnormal head posture would separate the diplopia by increasing the angle of squint.

Vertical palsies. A more complicated abnormal head posture occurs in these cases because the actions of the defective muscle are more complicated (Fig. 20). The head posture must counteract the secondary as well as the primary action of these muscles and thus it is seen to consist of three components.

1. Chin elevated or depressed, to compensate for the defective main action of the muscle.
2. Face turned to the right or left side to avoid the position of maximum influence of the main action.
3. Head tilted to the right or left shoulder to counteract the torsional and vertical results of the palsy. When the head is tilted it is physiological that torsion should occur to retain the upright position of the vertical meridian of the globe. Thus, if the head is tilted to the left shoulder, the left eye will become intorted and the right eye extorted. In addition, a tilt to one side will elevate the eye on the side of the tilt, and depress the other eye. The torsion which causes difficulty may either be due to the defective action of the paresed muscle or to the excessive action of the contralateral synergist. It should be remembered that the torsional power of the obliques is superior to that of the recti, and frequently the head tilt is in consideration of this fact, whether the oblique be the defective or the over-acting muscle.

Take, for example, a case of right superior rectus palsy.

1. The chin should be elevated because the main action is elevation, and by elevating the chin, a depressed position of the eyes is achieved.
2. The turn should be to the right since the main action of elevation

has greatest effect when the eye is abducted and, by turning the head to the right, the right eye is adducted.

3. The tilt may be to the right shoulder because the palsy will have resulted in excessive action of the left inferior oblique (the contralateral synergist) and its torsional action will have resulted in extorsion of the left eye which may demand a head tilt to the right to compensate for it; also, this tilt will to some extent compensate for the depression of the right eye. Alternatively, but rarely, the tilt may be to the left shoulder because the defective secondary action of the right superior rectus (intorsion) may have resulted in right extorsion, and this head tilt renders right extorsion physiological.

In the case of an oblique palsy there is not this possibility of a variation; for example, in a palsy of the right superior oblique there should be:

1. Depression of the chin, because the muscle's main action is depression, and by this means the eyes are elevated.
2. A turn to the left since the main action of depression has greatest effect when the eye is adducted, and by turning the head to the left the right eye will be abducted.
3. A tilt towards the left shoulder, because the right superior oblique should intort the eye and its palsy results in right extorsion. With this head tilt right extorsion is physiological. In addition, this tilt will, to some extent, compensate for the elevation of the right eye.

While it is certainly true to say that these are the general principles of an abnormal head posture in vertical palsy, it is also true that many cases show postures which do not entirely conform with the typical pattern but which, nevertheless, achieve the purpose of compensation.

The abnormal head posture is usually subconscious and is only likely to occur in cases with a palsy of a mild enough nature to enable binocular single vision to be maintained in part of the field of vision, the abnormal head posture transferring that area of single vision to a more convenient position. If binocular single vision cannot be achieved in any part of the field the patient will have no reward from the adoption of an abnormal head posture, and it is unlikely to develop. Exceptions are cases troubled by diplopia which is close together, but not close enough to join; these patients may adopt a posture which contrasts with those described above and which relieves symptoms by increasing the size of the squint and forcing the two images further apart.

An abnormal head posture incorporating a head tilt, which has been adopted from infancy in order to compensate for a congenital palsy of a vertically acting muscle, is known as an ocular torticollis, and this condition can lead to permanent abnormal curvatures of the spinal column if left untreated.

7

Visual acuity and amblyopia

The development of visual acuity requires not only normal anatomical structures but also normal visual experience for its reinforcement, and that this is particularly important during the early years of life is becoming increasingly clear. The developmental period of the eyes has been classically described as 'up to 7 or 8 years of age', but all the evidence now indicates that there is a much earlier acutely sensitive period which is certainly under 4 years of age and is likely to be before the age of two or two and a half, during which visual functions are fast developing.

It is obvious that good, and preferably equal, visual acuity in each eye is a pre-requisite for proper binocular co-ordination: it follows that an accurate assessment of visual acuity is an essential part of the investigation of any squint, while the correction of any visual defect and the prevention of any further deterioration are an essential preliminary to its treatment.

MEASUREMENT OF VISUAL ACUITY

The visual acuity should normally be tested for near and distance with and without glasses if worn. Each eye is effectively occluded while the other is tested; if this induces latent nystagmus monocular tests give unrealistic results and acuity should also be tested with both eyes open.

Adults and older children. Snellens test type for distance and the standard near type are used. It is important to use more than one test type so that different letters are presented to either eye; when testing for near the patient can read the letters from left to right with one eye and from right to left with the other. It is amazing how, anxious to please, a child can recite from memory as far as 6/24 with an eye capable only of counting fingers. Linear type should be used rather than single optotype tests in order to detect the crowding phenomenon (p. 66).

Aged three years and over. By the age of three years the average child can perform the Sheridan Gardiner matching letter test using the seven-letter pointing card with reliable accuracy, and the very intelligent child succeeds even younger. (It is also a very useful test for the illiterate and less severely handicapped). Again single optotypes should be avoided in routine testing, since linear type might reveal the presence of the crowding phenomenon (p. 66); for the reason the child should be taught to use the pointer card in conjunction with the Snellens test type rather than the single-letter booklet as soon as possible. Testing the 'good' eye first can give a hesitant child the confidence which comes with success and also reassures the examiner that the patient really does understand what to do. A different series of letters would then of course be used for the eye suspected of having the poorer visual acuity.

Eighteen months and over. The difficulties of testing the very young child can be overcome by various simple techniques; the alert child of eighteen months will respond to games involving matching toys or shapes and can identify easy pictures of graded size (Stycar set, Ffooks symbols, Beale-Collins pictures, etc.). It may be necessary to teach the test at close quarters at first, but once understood, it should be performed at the full 6 metres distance.

Firm total occlusion of each eye in turn while doing these tests is essential for reliable assessment and with good parental co-operation this can be introduced gradually as the 'game' proceeds—though until the child gains confidence, mother's hand may be the only method of occlusion tolerated. Marked protest at the covering of one eye and not of the other indicates the presence of unequal vision.

Under eighteen months. For these infants and for the shy or less able child, there are several methods of objective assessment.

The cover test (p. 18) can reveal much even where there is no obvious manifest squint, but the test must be done deftly and rapidly before attention is lost. It should be performed with an easily interchangeable series of small attractive fixation targets and the test is conducted with, in this case, a firm and friendly covering hand rather than an alarming occluder. The infant with good binocular single vision and good visual acuity tends to protest whichever eye is covered, whereas the child who shows definite resentment at cover of one eye but passively accepts cover of the other always has reduced vision in that eye.

Opto-kinetic nystagmus, used as an indication of the threshold of good vision, can be excited by horizontal movement of striped ribbons or scarves and by rotating striped drums of various design. A similar effect can be induced by the Catford drum, which is perhaps the most convenient instrument for this purpose. A gradually reducing size of steadily moving target can be presented first binocularly and then monocularly so that, with expertise, it is possible to establish the degree of near visual response in each eye.

Rolling white balls of graded size at given distance against a standard background, or presented on invisible wires from behind a black screen, may yield further information.

Tiny edible balls, such as 'hundreds and thousands' are picked up by most infants with little encouragement; it is generally done with the tips of the fingers and thumb if the child can distinguish individual balls, but involves clumsy groping if not seen separately; the difference is quite distinctive and is said to indicate a near visual acuity of 6/12 where successful.

Early diagnosis of visual disturbance is the key to the successful treatment of the defect and to the prevention of secondary complications. It therefore cannot be sufficiently stressed that the practical difficulties of investigating an infant must be approached with patience and persistence.

Further investigations

Stereograms discernable only when there is good visual acuity in each eye and good binocular single vision are very helpful where it is necessary to prove normality, as in routine child health visual screening or developmental checks, and for this purpose random-dot stereograms (p. 87), such as the TNO series, can be usefully employed.

There is a variety of possible reasons for a defective visual acuity and if either a unilateral or a bilateral reduction is revealed on testing the vision, the cause must be further investigated. This will entail ophthalmoscopic examination (under anaesthesia if necessary for the very young) to detect any possible pathological cause—the procedure and possible findings are both beyond the scope of this book. The two conditions typically associated with squint are refractive errors and amblyopia.

REFRACTIVE ERRORS

Refraction under mydriatic should be checked routinely if there is any doubt about a child's visual capabilities, even when 'good' distance visual acuity has been demonstrated; hypermetropia which does not impair the distance vision can be a real barrier to closework and may disturb the relationship between accommodation and convergence and lead to an accommodative squint. Opinions vary concerning how 'full' a correction is desirable for hypermetropia in the presence of a manifest convergent squint—some would prescribe what others would regard as an 'overcorrection'—but it is extremely important that a young child is given a clear, sharply defined retinal image at all distances and this must mean an accurate correction of errors, particularly astigmatism, and refraction checks at least once a year.

AMBLYOPIA

Amblyopia has been described as a reduction in vision for which no obvious cause is detected on clinical examination; the cause is almost invariably some interruption during early childhood of that clear and normal visual stimulus so necessary to reinforce the developing visual acuity.

In recent years animal experiments have considerably advanced our understanding of this: even short periods of partial or defocussed deprivation have been shown to prevent the development of the full visual potential of the deprived eye and clinical experience has demonstrated that the younger the child, the more rapidly is the vision lost—and there is no doubt that if amblyopia is not identified and treated promptly in the young child it may become intractable.

Deprivation of the visual stimulus may be partial (as in many forms of refractive error and in the deviating eye of childhood squint) or total, as in the bandaged eye and in conditions such as congenital cataract.

Classification

There are four principle types of amblyopia:

Stimulus deprivation amblyopia. This is a condition of reduced visual acuity resulting from interruption of form (foveal) and light (retinal) stimulus following any prolonged monocular deprivation during the early years of the developmental period.

Strabismus amblyopia. In the presence of a unilateral squint, although there is light stimulus, there is form deprivation owing to the fact that the fovea of the deviating eye receives an image other than that received by the fovea of the fixing eye. This image will be blurred because the (binocular) accommodation exerted is governed by the requirements of the fixing eye.

Anisometropic amblyopia. The inequality of the refractive errors results in a blurred image in one eye and consequent failure of visual acuity to develop. Because peripheral fusion is strong there is no manifest squint, so that such cases are frequently not detected until school eye tests take place, by which time very serious central amblyopia may have become established.

Ametropic amblyopia. The result, usually, of marked astigmatism, this is often bilateral, but only one meridian in either eye may be involved, so that it is sometimes called meridional amblyopia.

Investigation

Amblyopia may be diagnosed if, after excluding any pathological cause and correcting any refractive error, there is still a reduced visual acuity. However there are certain additional investigations which can be helpful.

The crowding phenomenon. It is a frequent characteristic of amblyopia that the visual acuity tested with a single optotype may be two or even more lines better than if tested with a linear type such as Snellens test type, when the contours of one letter overlap and blurr those of its neighbour. The cause is debated and its presence has no prognostic significance, but it is important to realise that visual acuity should be tested with linear test types to be certain of detecting all cases of amblyopia, since the single-optotype achievement may be satisfactory and misleading (differences as extreme as 6/6 with single optotype and 6/60 with linear test have been recorded).

A pin-hole. This device can be used with enormous advantage to demonstrate whether a reduced visual acuity is due to a refractive error or to some other cause—if the former, the visual deficiency is corrected by the pin-hole and in the case of amblyopia it is not. The patient should hold the pin-hole disc himself in order to 'find' the hole and meanwhile the other eye is, of course, occluded.

Contrast sensitivity. The ability to discriminate contours is also affected by the presence of amblyopia, and this function, recognised as important in enhancing visual acuity, can be measured by such devices as Arden's book of contrast sensitivity gratings.

Neutral density filters. In the event of any doubt about the diagnosis of amblyopia, neutral density filters can be used to distinguish between organic and functional visual loss, the visual acuity in the former condition being significantly reduced by the filters.

Visually evoked response. Electro-diagnostic tests such as the visually evoked response (VER) system may be the only way of assessing visual and possibly binocular potential where a pathological defect prevents normal ocular tests.

Uniocular fixation

A combination of several tests will give a clear diagnosis.

The cover test. Utilising the position of the corneal reflection when the fixing eye is covered can give an approximate idea of the state of uniocular fixation. It should be remembered that this is a crude method of diagnosing fixation, but it may be the only method available in children too young for assessment with a fixation ophthalmoscope. If the child is very restless a plaster occlusion may have to be put for a few moments over each eye in turn while watching how steadily he can fix the light. The result of assessing fixation by this method would be recorded as follows:

Fixation centric on gross examination. When the fixing eye is covered the movement of the deviating eye is consistent with the angle of squint, and the position of its corneal reflection is comparable with that in the fixing eye.

Eccentric fixation absolute on gross examination. No movement of the deviating eye to take up fixation when the fixing eye is covered; the corneal reflection is grossly displaced compared with that of the fixing eye.

Eccentric fixation non-absolute but steady on gross examination. There is a movement of the deviating eye to take up fixation when the fixing eye is covered, but fixation is still eccentric; the corneal reflection is displaced as compared with that in the fixing eye.

Fixation eccentric but unsteady on gross examination. There is a continuous searching movement of the deviating eye when the fixing eye is covered; the corneal reflection is always displaced as compared with the fixing eye.

The visuscope and the projectoscope. These are both modified ophthalmoscopes incorporating a diamond-shaped silhouette in the centre of the beam of light and they are the ideal and only truly accurate way of diagnosing fixation. (A simple attachment for an ophthalmoscope is also available.) The principle of the test is to ask the patient to fix the diamond while the examiner notes the position of its shadow on the fundus. It will fall on the fovea in normal cases, but if there is an anomaly of fixation the diamond will fall on a point of the retina other than the fovea.

Use varies from that of the ophthalmoscope in certain respects; the routine procedure is set out below.

1. Dilation of the pupils is by no means always necessary.
2. Always occlude the eye which is not being examined to ensure proper fixation by the eye being investigated.
3. First examine the eye judged to be normal by asking the patient to look at the diamond. This is to show the patient what is expected of him (he may have very great difficulty in seeing the diamond with the amblyopic eye) and also to show the examiner what the patient's normal fixation is like. A proportion of patients show a very unsteady foveal fixation, even in a normally-sighted eye and it could lead to erroneous conclusions if the squinting eye only were investigated.

4. Transfer the occlusion to the normal eye and ask the patient to fix the diamond with the amblyopic eye. There is often a time-lag before he finds the diamond due to the reduced acuity, but when he claims to be looking at it, the position of the shadow should be noted. To ensure real fixation ask the child to count the points or whether he sees a spot in the middle of the diamond (perhaps called, for a child, 'the star'), in order to engage his attention on the silhouette.

The situation diagnosed in this way may be (a) *centric fixation*—the star being fixed by the fovea or (b)*eccentric fixation*—the star being fixed by a point other than the fovea which may be parafoveal (within macular border), paramacular (adjacent to macular border) or peripheral. The fixation at this point may be steady or unsteady. (c) *No fixation demonstrable*—in which no definite area of fixation is preferred. Small degrees of very fine nystagmus are sometimes evident only on visuscope examination.

5. Finally, in the event of any but central fixation, the examiner should ask the patient to 'look ahead' in the usual way for ophthalmoscopic investigation while he objectively places the shadow of the diamond on to the fovea. The patient is then instructed to look at the diamond and, if the anomalous fixation is but weakly developed, he may momentarily retain the foveal fixation with which he has been presented.

A visuscope or projectoscope examination should be carried out on all cases of amblyopia before occlusion treatment is begun. It is possible to check the fixation of remarkably small children because even a placid 2-year-old will fix 'the star' simply because, with the other eye occluded, there is nothing else to look at while an even younger infant will consistently adjust his eye in relation to the star, so that any preference for non-foveal fixation becomes evident. It should be remembered that all subjective tests should be completed before this investigation since it leaves a mild after-image which would interrupt clinical tests.

The record of fixation anomalies is made clearer by the use of a sketch diagram of the fundus on which is marked the point or area used for fixation, coupled with a comment on its steadiness.

Past-pointing. This, when associated with eccentric fixation, is a phenomenon in which the adaptation of visual direction is incomplete. In cases of long-standing eccentric fixation the eccentric point has developed the projectional value of the fovea (i.e. straight-ahead). If this development is incomplete, the eccentric point has neither its original projectional value nor that of the fovea so that, when fixation is attempted with the affected eye, there is a false assessment of the position of the fixation object. Thus if the patient is asked to touch the object, he fails to do so.

If eccentric fixation is present, this test should be carried out and it should be stated whether past-pointing is demonstrable or not demonstrable; this gives information as to the fixity of the eccentric fixation.

Prognosis

Prognosis in amblyopia rests mainly on a balance of four factors, each of which may strongly influence the conclusion.

The refractive error of the amblyopic eye is, of course, of importance since in the presence of a gross refractive error good visual acuity may never be achieved. Anisometropia is also a problem, although it may be noted that children can tolerate a large difference in the optical correction of the two eyes—as much as eight dioptres—without experiencing aniseikonia.

The present age of the patient is of paramount importance. Amblyopia has been found to be most susceptible to treatment up to the age of 29 months, it recovers reasonably quickly in most children under 5 years, more slowly between 5 and 7 years, but after 8 years of age it is a tedious process. It cannot be overemphasised that rapid identification and referral for treatment prevents the development of serious amblyopia, which is to say that the period prior to treatment for any case of squint (or any suspected visual difficulty) should always be as short as possible. However, it would be foolish to quote an upper age limit when improvement is no longer a practical possibility; anisometropic amblyopes given glasses for the first time in their teens often respond to treatment and adults, forced to use an amblyopic eye by losing the other, have been known to make remarkable, if painstaking, progress.

It must be remembered, that if amblyopia is overcome in a patient over approximately 8 years of age who has a squint and has lost the power to fuse, permanent pathological diplopia may well result. A careful prognosis for the squint must also be made, therefore, before embarking on treatment for older patients.

The state of fixation is also of extreme significance. A visual acuity of 6/6 is only possible at the fovea, so that any eccentricity of fixation will inevitably reduce the visual acuity attained. Thus any departure from steady central fixation is an added factor against a good prognosis.

To dislodge eccentric fixation is easier the younger the patient, the less steady the fixation at the eccentric point and the further that point is from the macula.

Co-operation from patient, parent, schoolteacher and nursery school helper is absolutely essential; unless the prescribed glasses are worn and the recommended treatment carried out, success is unlikely and younger children certainly need parental interest and supervision when carrying out any 'homework exercises' (p. 77) which may be part of the treatment.

Although these are the factors with the strongest influence on the prognosis, there are other considerations which should also be taken into account.

The age of onset is significant because it pinpoints the stage which normal development of visual acuity had reached prior to its interruption by the squint. This is the 'point of arrest' and it is generally agreed that visual acuity can always be restored to this level at a later date, although further development depends on other factors. (It must, of course, be realised that the age at which the squint was first noticed is not necessarily the true age of onset.)

The duration of squint indicates the period during which the visual acuity has decreased as a result of amblyopia. It should be possible to reverse this 'amblyopia of extinction' within the limits set by the present age.

Previous treatment should be taken into account in view of the fact that the prognosis worsens as the patient grows older and therefore results not achieved by well-conducted treatment in the past are less likely to be achieved later.

The successful eradication of amblyopia is a very important part of squint treatment. For cases in which binocular single vision is to be restored it is an essential preliminary since sound binocular vision must be based on equal monocular vision; in cases of children for whom binocular single vision is not attained the standard of discharge should include equal visual acuity, albeit accompanied by the facultative suppression characteristic of an alternating squint. However, in patients over approximately 8 years of age who lack the ability to fuse the two monocular images, the danger of permanent pathological diplopia must not be forgotten and treatment should be approached with caution.

Management

The aim of treatment for amblyopia of any form is to gain the maximum visual acuity possible in the affected eye but, during the sensitive developmental period, the effect of treatment which imposes further deprivation of stimulus on the developing binocular visual system must be taken into consideration, and the minimum of occlusion followed by early surgical re-alignment of the visual axes is desirable. Among older children for whom there is little chance of binocular vision it may be wise to establish alternation of the squint—that is, a situation in which the child has no particular preference for one eye, but uses either according to convenience; often the left eye is preferred for the right field and vice versa in the presence of a convergent squint. This state of affairs obviously reduces the likelihood of the amblyopia recurring.

A number of forms of treatment have been devised and individual therapists will develop their skills in certain preferred methods. The commonest of these are occlusion and penalisation and the practicalities of carrying out these two types of treatment is described at the close of this chapter. However, the principles governing the management of amblyopia can be considered in more general terms: the need for early diagnosis of any form of amblyopia is plainly of paramount importance and the management and method of treatment depends largely on the age at which the defect is diagnosed and on the state of fixation in the affected eye.

Non-central fixation
This condition takes time to develop and is not, therefore, normally found in either young children or patients for whom treatment is started soon after the onset of a squint. However, it prevents the re-development of good visual acuity and if it is diagnosed the first step in the management must be its replacement by foveal fixation. This is attempted by a variety of methods depending on the details of the case concerned.

Occlusion. In all cases of eccentric fixation a trial period of total occlusion of the fixing eye is advisable. This period must not be longer than a week and some insist on a maximum of only three days before re-assessment with the visuscope. This occlusion may result in one of the following:

1. Central fixation is restored, in which case total occlusion of the normally fixing eye can be continued, as in patients who originally had central fixation.
2. There is a shift of the eccentric point. If this occurs, occlusion of the normally fixing eye should continue until either central fixation is established or the eccentric point seems static. These patients should be seen at weekly intervals and if they do not regain central fixation they should be treated as group 3 below.
3. The eccentric point remains static. These cases should be treated by constant, total occlusion worn on the face over the amblyopic

eye in order to prevent any further stimulus of the eccentric point and to dislodge gradually the eccentric fixation. The case should be reviewed at monthly intervals for re-assessment with the visuscope and treatment must be continued until the eccentric fixation is completely disrupted. This may take a period of as long as six months or more, but will be recognised by an aimless, wandering loss of fixation when the visuscope test is attempted. Not often is foveal fixation established without some period of exposure of that eye to light stimulus.

At this time the occlusion is reversed for a very short trial; some orthoptists prefer to keep the child in the hospital for an hour or two in order to re-check the fixation before allowing a longer trial of one or two days of occlusion at home. This moment of the reversal of the occlusion is a very critical one, and it is essential that the patient is not allowed to re-establish the eccentric fixation he has so painstakingly lost. Once foveal fixation is confidently established, management proceeds as in central fixation described below.

Failure to disrupt eccentric fixation by occlusion will prevent the re-development of a good visual acuity. However, where pleoptic treatment (p. 73) is not advised, occlusion of the normally fixing eye can be carried out to get maximum visual acuity at the eccentric point but the practical and psychological difficulties of this treatment are great and careful assessment of each case is important.

Eccentric fixation in large angled squints may respond better to the occlusion management described above after surgery has been carried out to reduce the size of the deviation.

Inverse prism. Treatment by a combination of totally occluding the fixing eye and placing an inverse prism before the deviating eye is advocated by some ('inverse' in that a base-in prism is used for a convergent deviation). It has the effect of forcing the eye into the 'straight ahead' position as the patient takes up his eccentric fixation through the prism; his localisation of the fixation object is thus disturbed. It has been found by experience that the power of the prism should lie between $6^{\triangle}$ and $20^{\triangle}$ (even for a deviation which theoretically requires more) because this is sufficient to bring the eye close enough to 'straight' to encourage the fovea to attain the principal visual direction. Supervision of this method of treatment has to be very meticulous and detailed.

Penalisation. A form of drug penalisation (p. 76) is another suggested method of treating eccentric fixation; atropine drops 1.00 per cent are prescribed for the fixing eye and phosphaline iodide drops 0.06 per cent for the deviating eye, so that the patient uses the unaffected eye for distance and the amblyopic one for near. Excellent results are claimed for this method.

Red filter method. This is another approach to the problem. By this means only light to which cones are sensitive reaches the retina so that peripheral fixation, involving rods, is prohibited. The requisite filter is the Kodak No. 92 or the more serviceable Ruby Kodaloid and it is clipped onto the glasses in front of the eccentrically fixing eye, the other being totally occluded with plaster on the face. This type of occlusion can only be carried out for limited periods each day under supervision and, when not being worn, the eccentrically fixing eye is occluded. Results prove satisfactory in some cases after an initial period of total occlusion of the eccentrically fixing eye.

Pleoptic treatment. Certain selected cases which have not responded to occlusion therapy may be considered for pleoptic treatment. It must be accompanied by constant total occlusion on the face over the amblyopic eye and involves daily attendance at the clinic for a period of several weeks with frequent attendance afterwards. Because of this serious interruption to schooling or to work, careful selection for treatment is necessary, bearing in mind the fact that abnormal retinal correspondence is almost invariably revealed once the fixation has been centralised, and that the chances of binocular single vision being restored are negligible and so, if treatment is lightly undertaken, there is a very real risk that insuperable diplopia will result.

However, in monocular patients there is no doubt that pleoptic treatment can improve visual acuity in many cases which would otherwise have to be regarded as 'intractable' and in this field it can be of enormous value.

Skill and experience are necessary if pleoptic treatment is to be successfully conducted. It is not in the everyday experience of the average ophthalmologist or orthoptist and those wishing to undertake it are referred to the wide literature available and, if possible, are advised to receive personal tuition in an established pleoptic clinic.

Central fixation

If central fixation is already present, treatment of amblyopia is by occlusion (p. 75) of the normally fixing eye in order to promote the use of the amblyopic eye or by penalisation (p. 76) of the fixing eye by lenses or drugs so that the visual acuity of that eye is sufficiently reduced to stimulate the use of the other one. In all cases the age of the patient is a strongly decisive factor in planning the management; this is mainly because the patients in the younger groups should not be subjected to prolonged total deprivation of visual stimulus unless imperative for other reasons, since they are still within the highly sensitive developmental period.

A rare condition found occasionally in children under about 5 years of age is 'switch' or occlusion amblyopia, when the occluded eye has become amblyopic (possibly even to the point of fixing eccentrically) after a brief period of occlusion. This is increasingly uncommon in patients over about 3, but patients of any age who are having treatment for amblyopia should always be checked frequently to see that the form and intensity of treatment advised is indeed the best for that particular individual.

Infant cases. In its very early stages, strabismus amblyopia in unilateral squint from birth or early infancy can be prevented or corrected by judicious short periods (as little as five minutes) cover of the fixing eye during waking hours. A soft eye pad is a suitable occlusion, but even the mother's hand held carefully over the fixing eye can be used to start with.

The 'toddler'. Occlusion for between 20 and 60 minutes daily can be used for this age group and an elastoplast occluder or an extension fitted onto the glasses, if worn, will be required. Sitting on the mother's knee looking at picture books for some period while wearing the occlusion will hasten the treatment.

The three-year-old. By the age of 3 it is often possible to encourage total occlusion for up to about two hours daily and closework tasks while occluded are very desirable. Total occlusion for short periods is preferable to longer periods of partial occlusion for this age group since long interruptions to visual stimulus are suspected of having an adverse effect on the young visual system. Drug penalisation (p. 76) may be helpful with its twin advantages of being a form of partial deprivation and requiring no co-operation from the child in tolerating a patch; however, it should be used as a last resort in this age group since it cannot be discontinued quickly in the event of switch amblyopia.

Between four and seven years of age. In this age group longer periods of occlusion may be introduced routinely; by school age prolonged total occlusion will be needed to make any impact on firmly established amblyopia and penalisation may also be effective. There is a belief that the occlusion period can be for as little as seven minutes daily while stimulated with the Cambridge vision stimulator (the 'Cam'), but while many would consider this too brief, there is no doubt that increasingly it is felt that the secret of successful occlusion treatment is not so much the length of time each day during which the occlusion is worn, as the amount of concentrated closework which is attempted while it is worn. The actual period of the day chosen for occluding is therefore most important, and meal time, out-of-doors time and even television time are not as effective as during concentrated activities such as colouring pictures or playing with jig saw puzzles or when doing school homework.

Over the age of eight. In selecting cases for treatment over the age of 8 it must be remembered that, if no fusion is present, irreversible pathological diplopia could be the outcome of eliminating the suppression which accompanies amblyopia. Treatment of older patients should, therefore, be limited to those with intermittent squints or in whom the potential power to fuse is demonstrably strong. Regular checks for the first signs of pathological diplopia should be made and treatment must be discontinued if there is any danger of this permanent and distressing symptom. For this reason drug penalisation is not very wise for this group of patients, because of the period of time which must elapse after the drug has been discontinued before its effect has worn off.

Amblyopia treatment is slow in older patients, but there can be a very rewarding improvement in visual acuity among monocular adult cases when the amblyopic eye is forced into use, through injury or disease affecting the hitherto fixing eye. Pleoptic (p. 73) and other forms of intensive foveal stimulation (p. 78) have been known to restore virtually normal sight in adults with long standing gross amblyopia.

Methods of treatment
The two most common forms of treatment for amblyopia are occlusion and penalisation and there are several ways in which each of these methods of treatment can be varied to suit individual cases.

Occlusion
A method of treatment whereby one eye is covered in order to encourage the use of the other eye. The degree by which the visual acuity of the covered eye is obscured can be very finely adjusted by selecting the particular form of occlusion appropriate to the situation. Any one patient may progress through several variations during the course of treatment.

Total occlusion. This either results in total deprivation of light and form stimulus or it allows light to enter the eye but prevents the formation of an image.

Complete plaster occlusion. The patch is made from three-inch porous elastoplast with a protecting central lining of lint and is worn stuck to the face; it thus excludes light as well as preventing the formation of an image. Its advantages are that it is difficult for a small child to peep round it and it is unquestionably more effective than other forms of total occlusion. Its disadvantages are the discomfort it involves and the fact that a small child's skin may not tolerate it for long.

Extension occlusion. The next alternative is to attach an occlusion to the spectacle frame; this may be made in the clinic with washable zinc oxide plaster or micropore and a commercially produced one which clips onto the spectacles is obtainable. The occlusion extends to meet the brow and cheek and forms a blinker down the side of the glasses so that light is virtually excluded. It is unquestionably pleasanter for the patient to wear than adhesive plaster occlusion, but it demands more co-operation because it is very easy to peep momentarily over the top whenever really sharp visual acuity is required.

Lens occlusion. Such treatment may be carried out by sticking adhesive paper, plaster, blenderm or music mending paper to the spectacle lens and again calls for co-operation from the patient who must realise that he is not allowed to peep.

Partial occlusion. This allows the formation of an image but diminishes the visual acuity of the occluded eye. This type of occlusion is used as the visual acuity of the amblyopic eye approaches that of the usually-fixing eye and it can be graded to render the visual acuity of the two eyes equal. It is also used to eliminate small degrees of amblyopia in cases maintaining binocular single vision.

Translucent adhesive tape. Several well-known brands are marketed and they are extremely useful. It does not wash off, is quickly replaced and may be graded by varying the number of layers prescribed.

Colourless nail varnish. This is useful in that it can be stippled by a brush to the degree of opacity required. Care must be taken that frames (or lenses, if plastic) are not damaged by the remover.

Commercially produced occlusions. Again, these are usually graded to permit a particular visual acuity.

Atropine. This is sometimes used if occlusion is not possible either because the skin is too sensitive or because the patient constantly pulls it off (and it may also be used as part of a penalisation regime). Atropine ointment 1 per cent is instilled daily in the usually-fixing eye and if glasses are being worn it is sensible temporarily to remove the lens before the normal eye, leaving the amblyopic one corrected.

Penalisation

The term penalisation indicates a form of treatment which forces the patient to use one eye for distance and the other for near by means of lenses and/or drugs. The first stage of the treatment is to develop the near visual acuity in the amblyopic eye by penalising the fixing eye for near, and then moving on to develop distance visual acuity by preventing the unaffected eye from seeing clearly in the distance.

Near penalisation. Each day throughout treatment 1.0 per cent atropine is instilled into the fixing eye while a Fresnel lens of strength varying between +1.50DS and +4.00DS is added to the spectacle lens before the amblyopic eye. The patient, while still able to use the normally fixing eye for distance, is thus prevented from using it for near, so that the amblyopic eye is forced to take up near fixation.

Near penalisation may also be achieved by prescribing 1.0 per cent atropine each morning for the unaffected eye and 0.06 per cent phospholine iodide each evening for the amblyopic eye.

Distance penalisation. The atropinised fixing eye is handicapped for distance by a Fresnel +3.00DS which allows clear near vision, while the amblyopic eye has no atropine and merely the normal refractive correction. The amblyopic eye is thus forced into use for distance vision, and may also be used for near—the near vision having recently been encouraged by near penalisation.

Total penalisation. This is not, strictly speaking, a true form of penalisation as the visual acuity of the normally fixing eye is, in effect, so handicapped that the amblyopic eye is forced into use for both near and distance. The fixing eye is limited by an instillation of 1.0 per cent atropine daily coupled with a Fresnel −4.00DS or −5.00DS lens thus making clear vision for both near and distance impossible. The amblyopic eye is prescribed a full refractive correction and, in some instances, placed in a condition of miotic-induced myopia with the use of phospholine iodide 0.06 per cent each evening.

Discussion. The nature and degree of penalisation is determined by altering the ratio of the drugs and lenses, and variations of the principle are found in different hospitals. The advantages over conventional occlusion include the fact that at no time is there deprivation of light stimulus to either eye, it is less conspicuous, there is no chance of the patient peeping round a patch so that the child's active co-operation is not required, and there is no aggravation of latent nystagmus. Disadvantages include the long-term use of drugs (although no worrying side affects are reported in the literature), the long time-lag between discontinuing the use of drugs and the end of their influence, so that treatment cannot be abruptly discontinued, and the twice-daily instillations which children often do not enjoy.

Visual excercises

Experience has shown that the value of both occlusion and penalisation is greatly increased by considering definite daily periods of meticulous closework using the amblyopic eye as part of the treatment. Small children can be encouraged to identify detail in nursery pictures and colour-in black and white illustrations, while older children can draw 'dot-to-dot' pictures, trace and read, and all age groups play jig-saw puzzles. Watching television appears to have very little impact on the amblyopic eye and cannot be considered part of the therapy. If children are of school age, the teachers should understand that, while closework may not be up to standard during treatment, it should certainly not be discontinued.

Foveal stimulation

Recent experiments have greatly increased our knowledge of the physiology of vision and the aeteology of amblyopia. It has now been demonstrated that visual cells in the brain respond best to gratings of a particular size and orientation and a form of treatment has been devised at Cambridge which attempts to respond to this new knowledge by stimulating the amblyopic eye with gratings in all orientations. This is achieved by an instrument, the Cambridge vision stimulator (or the Cam) on which concentrated closework is carried out on a transparent plate, behind which is a disc of square-wave gratings of selected size which rotates at one revolution per minute, thus constantly altering the orientation of the gratings.

Total occlusion is worn over the normally fixing eye for seven minutes and the amblyopic eye is used with intense concentration in games and exercises devised for different age groups. First reports claim spectacular successes with an average of four daily treatments each lasting seven minutes, with no necessity to occlude the fixing eye between treatments.

Parental understanding

This is also of extreme importance not only to ensure that the child is properly supervised and the treatment carried out, but also to avoid unnecessary fears which can arise through inadequate explanation. The most common disappointment during occlusion treatment is that the eye is 'beautifully straight when the patch is on but goes back into the corner again as soon as it is taken off' and the fear that 'the squint has gone over into the good eye too' can arise if alternation occurs. Time must be found to make certain that parents understand at all stages the aim of the treatment advised.

Duration

It is difficult to predict how long treatment will be necessary, although in general the younger patients respond more rapidly than the older ones. The length of time taken to achieve an improvement from, say,

6/36 to 6/6 varies and is dependent not only on the occlusion or penalisation used but on the concurrent response to correction of any refractive error and possible squint surgery.

One month is usually allowed to elapse between appointments during the bulk of treatment (if co-operation is good) but shorter intervals are essential for those under 4 and where it is hoped to re-establish some form of binocular vision. Early recovery of binocular single vision obviously reduces the overall duration of treatment, but where this is not possible attendance must continue until either alternation prevents recurrence of amblyopia or, if uniocular fixation persists, until maximum visual acuity of the affected eye becomes stable. This latter course is the least satisfactory and may require careful monitoring for several years.

The role of the orthoptist
If the squinting patient is to have bi-foveal binocular single vision restored, a first essential is the elimination of amblyopia, while on the other hand, if the prognosis for a binocular result is poor, it is an advantage to the child if either eye is capable of a good visual acuity. This means that the diagnosis and treatment of amblyopia is an important part of the orthoptist's work. She is trained to assess the visual acuity in patients of all ages, to select the cases that will benefit from treatment, to plan the management and to undertake the most appropriate form of therapy. It is implicit in this that she is conscious of the patients for whom treatment could be harmful (either in the loss of binocular vision during the sensitive period, or in eliciting pathological diplopia or in disturbing the binocular function of a patient with an intermittent squint) and will take the precautions necessary to avoid these outcomes.

8

Investigation of squint

A full investigation of a manifest squint should, of course, seek to
reveal not only the direction and size of the deviation, but also the
extent to which the squint may have affected the visual and binocular
functions, the muscular balance and the posture of the patient. The
cover test, to determine the direction of the squint, has already been
described and, after a discussion of the various means of measuring
the size of the deviation, the methods of investigation will be
described in the sequence followed when describing the effects of
squint in Chapter 6. Finally some comments will be made regarding
the best clinical approach to the general investigation of cases of
squint and the modifications necessary when examining an infant.

MEASUREMENT OF THE DEVIATION

There are three principal methods of measuring a deviation, each with
its own advantages in different circumstances.

The major amblyoscope

This is the most common instrument used for the measurement of a
squint for it is ingenious in its simplicity and results may be obtained
from patients of as little as 2 years old.

Basically the instrument (Plate IV) consists of two cylindrical tubes
with a mirrored right-angle bend and containing in the eye-piece a
convex lens (Fig. 18). At the outer end of each tube there is a slide
carrier into which pictures are inserted (so that each eye is stimulated
by a separate image) and the total length of the tube is equal to the
focal length of the lens. Thus the emergent rays are parallel and no
accommodation is required by the patient. The tubes are supported
on columns in such a way that the pictures may be moved in relation
to each other horizontally, vertically and torsionally and each of these
adjustments is indicated on a series of scales. An account of the
additional refinements of the instrument is not necessary for the
present purpose and a detailed description of its handling is beyond
the scope of this book.

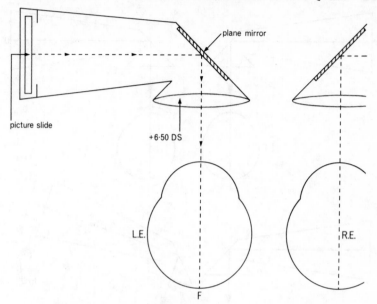

Fig. 18 Principles of the major amblyoscope

To measure the size of the angle of squint the cover test principle is employed. Two picture slides are inserted in the carriers and with the tubes set at 0° the patient is asked to look from one to the other while each picture in turn is illuminated. In the event of the visual axes being other than parallel there must be a movement of the deviating eye to take up foveal fixation of the picture presented to it (Fig. 19a).

By the same principle as the cover test an outward movement to take up fixation denotes a convergent deviation; the patient continues to look from picture to picture while the amblyoscope tube is rotated into the convergent position until no further movement of the eye to take up fixation is noted. The size of the deviation is then read from the scale, indicating the arc through which the tube has been moved. A convergent angle is designated + and a divergent angle − (Fig. 19b).

By the same method vertical and torsional adjustments can be made and, as the measurement is taken fixing with either eye and in all nine positions of gaze, inconcomitance can be accurately diagnosed.

While the major amblyoscope measurement is the simplest to carry out and has the advantage of enabling vertical and torsional elements of the deviation to be accurately assessed, it is true to say that horizontal inaccuracies may occur due to convergence accompanying the (unnecessary) accommodative effort patients often exert. Thus major amblyoscope readings may show a larger convergent or smaller divergent angle than is, in fact, the case.

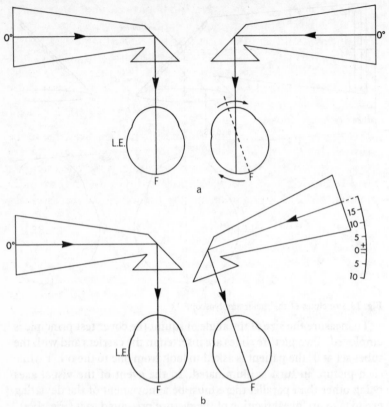

Fig. 19 Measurement of convergent squint

The prism cover test

In order to carry out this objective test and achieve an accurate assessment of the deviation, the patient must have central fixation and sufficient concentration to maintain steady fixation while the test is being carried out. The deviation can be measured at any distance, but normally the measurements are taken at one-third of a metre and at 6 metres with a light as fixation object, and at one-third of a metre with a fixation object which induces accommodation. The deviation can also be measured in the nine cardinal position of gaze. The patient is required to fix the target at the stated distance, and the strength of the prisms is increased while alternate eyes are covered by an opaque occluder. When there is no longer any movement of the eye on removal of the occluder, the maximum angle of deviation has been measured. The prism is placed base-out for a convergent deviation, base-in for a divergent deviation, base-up before a hypotropic eye and base-down before a hypertropic eye (see Plate III).

This test is carried out in natural conditions, and measures manifest and latent deviations without inducing unnecessary accommodation and thus gives the most accurate assessment of the deviation. It is really the only satisfactory method of measuring the deviation in intermittent squint where a comparison of near and distance deviations is required, e.g. convergent squint of the convergence excess type and intermittent divergent squint. It is also the best way when planning surgery.

However, large angles cannot be measured in this way due to the aberration caused by high prismatic powers and a deviation involving both horizontal and vertical elements is difficult for one examiner alone to measure, since two prism bars and the cover test occluder must all be held. In addition torsion cannot be compensated for prismatically.

Reflection assessment
It may be necessary simply to note reflex positions in cases with inadequate co-operation for other tests or in patients with gross amblyopia or eccentric fixation who are unable to take up foveal fixation to perform the dissociation methods of measurement. In all measurements by reflections the position of the corneal reflex on the fixing eye should first be noted since this gives an indication of the position of the patient's fovea in relation to the optic axis.

On the major amblyoscope. The tubes are adjusted until the corneal reflections of the two eyes are symmetrical.

By the prism reflection test. A torch is held in the near position and prisms are increased until the corneal reflections are symmetrical.

By Hirschberg's method. The deviation can be assessed by noting the position of the corneal reflex on the squinting eye. A torch is held in the near position and it is said that a reflex on the pupil margin is due to a squint of 10° to 15°, a reflex half way between the pupil margin and the limbus to one of 25° and a reflex on the limbus indicates a squint of approximately 45°. This method of assessment is ideal for infants, although only approximate as the pupil size is variable.

VISUAL TESTS

Visual acuity
This extremely important aspect of the investigation of all cases of squint has been described in detail in Chapter 7.

Pathological diplopia
In children pathological diplopia will probably only be found in cases of very recent or intermittent onset, but in adults it will persist for

long periods after the onset of squint, and may never be suppressed. Care should be taken to differentiate between pathological diplopia and blurring of the image—a distinction which may be missed by the patient.

Non-paretic squints

Pathological diplopia is not persistent in non-paretic squints. A child quickly suppresses and such squints rarely have an onset in adult life, except in cases of recently decompensated heterophoria. Investigation is simplest with Worth's lights, viewed through dissociating red and green goggles. The red and green lights are thus only visible to the eye behind the matching filter, and the white light, which is seen by both eyes, is converted by the filters to their colour. It is customary to place the red filter before the right eye and thus, in the presence of pathological diplopia, the right eye sees two red lights and the left eye sees three green ones. In convergent squints the pathological diplopia will be homonymous (or uncrossed) and the two red lights will be on the right of the three green ones. A divergent squint causes heteronymous (or crossed) pathological diplopia.

However, most patients with non-paretic squint have suppressed the squinting eye and will see only either two red or three green lights. (Binocular single vision is demonstrated with Worth's lights when a patient sees four lights, the bottom one being a fused mixture of red and green).

Paretic squints

Acquired paretic squints are usually accompanied by pathological diplopia. In a child suppression is slower in paretic than in non-paretic squint because the inconcomitance of the deviation results in varying retinal elements being stimulated; in an adult suppression is very rare indeed.

The investigation should open with questions regarding the frequency of the diplopia, whether there is any position in which it is joined and also in which position it is most widely separated. Finally the patient should be asked if the images are separated purely horizontally or if a vertical element is involved. A purely horizontal separation suggests a medial or lateral rectus palsy since any of the other muscles must affect the vertical balance. During the enquiry the patient's posture should be noted, as an abnormal head posture may have been adopted in order to join the diplopia.

Clinical investigation is carried out with red and green goggles (again worn, conventionally, with a red filter before the right eye) and the Armstrong Bar-lite attachment to a torch which converts the spot of light into a line. The patient's head must be straight and the torch is held vertically in each of the nine cardinal positions of gaze (commonly described as 'along the lines of the Union Jack') while the patient describes the relative position of the two lights. The variation in separation will be in accordance with the inconcomitance and thus the maximum separation will be seen when looking in the direction in which the main action of the paretic muscle has its greatest effect (pp. 95–98). In palsies of vertically acting muscles the greatest torsional effect will be at 90° to this direction. Furthermore, since in this direction the paretic eye will be limited in action, it follows from the principles of normal projection that the further image will be that seen by the paretic eye.

Thus, if maximum separation is noted on laevo-depression, the affected muscle will either be the left inferior rectus or the right superior oblique (since both have their main action at its maximum in this direction) and if the further image is red, it will be the right superior oblique (the red filter being before the right eye). The patient will however be aware of greatest torsional disturbance on dextro-depression, since it is here that the right superior oblique will be defective in its action of intorsion; the right eye will be extorted and the image, consequently, intorted.

It is possible to record the findings on a chart, laying out the relative position of the two images in all directions of gaze, but usually a simple recording of the position in which maximum separation is noted, coupled with a statement of which was the further image, is sufficient; this will pin-point the affected muscle. It is also important to record the presence, if any, of a direction in which diplopia does not occur.

The field of binocular fixation. If diplopia is not present in all directions of gaze this should also be charted. It is best done on the perimeter simply by asking the patient to watch the moving target as it is withdrawn from the centre on successive arcs of the field and to indicate the change from diplopia to single vision. This will chart the area over which binocular single vision is maintained, and is invaluable in long term observation as a record of change—and evidence of improvement can be a great source of comfort to an anxious patient. It is also an indication of the actual discomfort he is suffering. If a perimeter is not easily available for the orthoptist, fields of binocular fixation plotted on the Hess screen can be perfectly satisfactory.

Confusion

Patients very rarely notice this, owing to the extremely rapid suppression of the fovea which occurs after the onset of a squint. If it is present it requires no investigation.

Suppression

Pathological diplopia is, very commonly, suppressed. Its presence can be demonstrated clinically simply by the failure to elicit diplopia, but more detailed tests can be carried out on the major amblyoscope to define the areas and density of suppression. The importance of investigating suppression in adult cases for whom surgery is considered is described on page 130.

Amblyopia

This is said to be present if the ophthalmoscopic examination reveals no pathological cause, if any refractive error has been corrected and yet the visual acuity of one eye remains lower than it should be considering the age of the patient. The investigation has been described in Chapter 7.

Uniocular fixation. It is extremely important to examine the uniocular fixation of all cases showing diminished visual acuity and details of the investigation are given on pages 66 to 68.

BINOCULAR FUNCTION

When carrying out the visual tests, some indication of possible binocular function may have been gained, particularly if pathological diplopia is recognised, but more specific examination is now necessary.

Fusion

The power of fusion is the basis of the maintenance of binocular single vision and therefore it is essential in the diagnosis of a case of squint to investigate the fusion potential. This is in order, in a constant squint, to discover the lengths to which its degeneration through lack of use has gone and, in an intermittent squint, to discover what reserves of fusion there are to enable the re-establishment of constant binocular single vision.

Although there are several methods of demonstrating the presence of fusion and of exercising it, the only really competent method of assessing its potential strength in patients with a manifest squint is on the major amblyoscope. Two slides of a similar design are placed in the carriers and, if the tubes are in the correct position to compensate for the angle of squint, normal binocular conditions are simulated since each fovea is being presented with a similar image.

The clinical investigation of fusion is a skilful and important function of the orthoptist and the method will not be detailed here. It is sufficient to say that the orthoptist will determine whether the ability to fuse has survived the squinting period of monocular vision and she will also give a measure of the reserve of fusion. This is investigated by gradually adjusting the position of the two monocular images so that they no longer correspond with the exact position of the visual axes. If fusion is to be maintained the foveal position must be equally adjusted by the patient. The positive fusional reserve is measured by inducing convergence, and the negative reserve by inducing divergence.

Before fusion can be said truly to exist a small reserve must be demonstrable. For example, a patient with a convergent squint of 10° may superimpose the fusion slides with the instrument placed at +10° but if the images break apart as soon as convergence is attempted fusion cannot be said to be present. It is difficult to express a binding standard for the assessment of fusion, but approximately 5° of positive fusional range is necessary before the patient can be said to have fused—rather than superimposed—the images. Weak fusion may be diagnosed if the eyes can be converged 5° to 10° from the squinting angle, moderate fusion if 10° to 25° of positive range is demonstrable, and strong fusion if over 25° is easily attained. The normal negative fusional range (of approximately 5°) is too small to show accurate diagnostic differences but the normal positive fusional range is so large (approximately 45° to 50°) that shades of diagnostic significance are discernible.

Stereoscopic vision

Stereopsis can be investigated on the major amblyoscope, this time graded by the use of successively more difficult slides, and the Wirt stereo test is also a guide to the presence and extent of stereopsis. Random dot stereograms are easy to use and the disparate dot-patterns seen through red and green goggles in the TNO series are simple enough in character for even very young children to recognise. These tests have the enormous advantage of allowing no real opening for guessing and a similar advantage is found in the limitless variation of the Frisby stereotest (Plate V). Here a circular area can be discerned in depth within a field of flecked shapes printed on either side of plastic plates of varying thickness, thus producing disparate images.

Stereoacuity

The acuity of a patient's stereoscopic vision can be measured by recording the minimum disparity of the two monocular images which

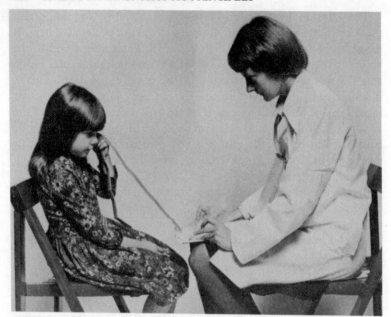

Plate V The Frisby stereotest

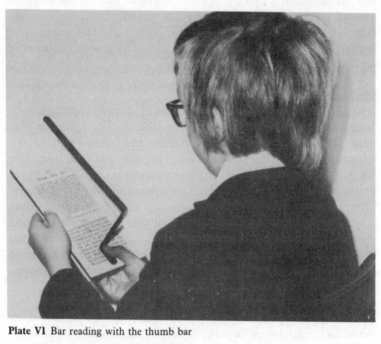

Plate VI Bar reading with the thumb bar

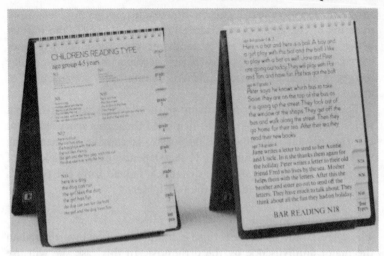

Plate VII The Maclure children's reading type and bar reading book

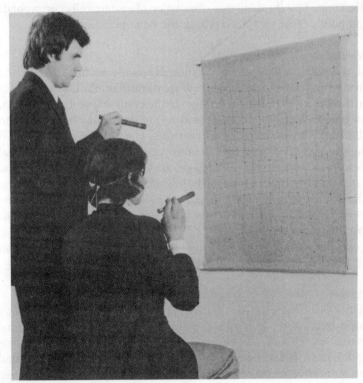

Plate VIII A simple Hess screen

results in stereoscopic recognition. Stereoacuity is therefore measured in terms of the angle of resolvable binocular disparity, the normal being considered to be 60 seconds of arc; those with weaker stereoacuity require greater disparity between the two monocular images and many young children demonstrate stereoacuity of approximately 240 secs.

The TNO test covers a range from 480 to 15 secs, achieving this by a series of individual test-patterns displaced through a specified arc at the test distance of 40 cm. The Frisby is capable of measuring stereoacuity ranging from 600 to 15 secs depending on the thickness of the plastic plate in use and the distance it is held from the patient's eyes—a tape is provided with the test folder.

Retinal correspondence

The correspondence of the retinae is another function investigated on the major amblyoscope by the orthoptist. In this case she will use totally dissimilar images for either eye (the classic example being the lion and the cage) and the correspondence between the retinae is determined by checking that stimulation of anatomically corresponding points results in projection to the same point in space.

Normal retinal correspondence

If the major amblyoscope is adjusted exactly to the angle of the manifest squint so that both foveae are stimulated, the lion will appear to the patient to be inside the cage. In the event of foveal suppression, an image stimulating a larger area of the retina may be required to illustrate the correspondence between the retinae. Therefore, if suppression prevents the demonstration of simultaneous foveal perception, parafoveal sized images are used and finally paramacular sized ones. In this way, the orthoptist will be able to specify whether the normal retinal correspondence is present as simultaneous foveal perception, simultaneous macular perception or simultaneous paramacular perception.

Lack of retinal correspondence. This will be diagnosed if suppression of either image persistently prevents their superimposition.

Abnormal retinal correspondence

Three principal tests—on the major amblyoscope, with Bielchowsky's after image test, and with Bagolini glasses—may reveal abnormal retinal correspondence; Worth's lights can also be used. The first is quick and effective in most cases, while the second and third depend on subjective responses which are rather complicated for a young patient to understand.

The major amblyoscope. This method is simply to measure the exact size of the squint first and then to discover if stimulation of the two foveae results in localisation to the same point in space—in other words, to discover if the lion appears to be in the cage when the instrument tubes are set at the angle of squint. If the patient insists that the lion is only in the cage when the tubes are at a lesser angle, it is apparent that the correspondence between the retinae is not strictly that of fovea-to-fovea.

An angle of anomaly is said to exist if there is a difference between the objectively measured angle, i.e. the actual angle of squint, and the subjective angle, i.e. the angle at which the patient reports superimposition of the two pictures. Thus if the angle of squint is +20° and the subjective angle is +12°; the angle of anomaly is 8°.

Abnormal retinal correspondence causes an angle of anomaly, as the fovea of one eye is used in conjunction with a peripheral retinal element of the other eye. This angle of anomaly increases as the abnormal retinal correspondence develops, until finally it equals the angle of squint in harmonious abnormal retinal correspondence.

There are other reasons for an angle of anomaly occurring and it is, therefore, an error to consider that all angles of anomaly are an indication of abnormal retinal correspondence.

Central suppression, which prevents the easy superimposition of the images, causes an unsteady angle of anomaly of 1° to 3°.

An accommodative element tends to cause an increase in convergence on prolonged fixation and results in a larger angle being demonstrated in the slightly longer objective test. This may be of any size from 2° to 20° but the experienced orthoptist recognises the characteristic hovering of the eyes in a patient with variable accommodation.

Bielchowsky's after image test. Retinal correspondence can also be demonstrated by after images. Each eye is successively exposed to a vivid flash of light in the form of a bar with a central unilluminated red spot which must be steadily fixed by the fovea during stimulation. The bar of light is placed horizontally before the usually fixing eye first and then vertically before the usually squinting eye. The patient is then instructed to close his eyes and is questioned on the resulting after-image. Since each fovea fixed the central spot in the bar, normal retinal correspondence will result in an after-image in the form of a cross thus $-\frac{1}{1}$ since the two foveae project to the same point in space. If, however, there is abnormal retinal correspondence the centres of the after-image bars will not be superimposed, but will be separated. In a case of right convergent squint it will appear thus $\frac{1}{1}--$ and in left convergent squint thus $--\frac{1}{1}$ since the squinting eye is stimulated with the vertical bar. Abnormal retinal correspondence is rare in divergent squint, but in a right divergent squint it would appear thus--¦ and in a left divergent squint thus¦--.

This test gives a different emphasis from the major amblyoscope in that it will not indicate abnormal retinal correspondence as long as traces of normal retinal correspondence remain, whereas the major amblyoscope will show abnormal responses in the early stages of its development.

The test is available in various forms, the two most commonly used being the electronic flash, which has an instantaneous effect owing to the brilliance of the light, and the adaptation of the major amblyoscope. This is slower in creating the after-image but may be followed by alternating light and dark phases which make the after-image more easily recognisable.

Striated glasses of Bagolini. Each glass consists of cylinders which will convert a source of light into a line in much the same way as a Maddox rod. By using a Bagolini glass in front of each eye, with the axes of the cylinders at right angles to each other, a St Andrew's cross may be seen when fixing a spotlight. Thus dissimilar objects are presented to each eye, but there is no dissociation by colour or cover so that the most natural conditions possible are retained; for that reason this is probably the most satisfactory test for diagnosing abnormal retinal correspondence.

If the patient has the harmonious type of abnormal retinal correspondence he will observe a symmetrical cross passing through the centre of the light, which proves that the fovea of one eye is being used in conjunction with an extra-macular point of the other eye. Should the two streaks of light not form a perfect cross the patient must have either inharmonious abnormal retinal correspondence or normal retinal correspondence, and now prisms equivalent to the angle of deviation must be used in order to diagnose the state of correspondence. They will result in bifoveal stimulation, so that if the correspondence is normal a perfect cross will of necessity be seen; if the correspondence is abnormal, the streaks of light will still not form a perfect cross, but will be displaced sideways.

Worth's lights are used and interpreted in the same way as Bagolini glasses but the visual stimulus of the four coloured dots is disturbed by colour dissociation, which is not always very satisfactory.

Other clinical characteristics. Patients with abnormal retinal correspondence have residual amblyopia of the squinting eye (approximately two lines less than the fixing eye) and, if any 'fusion' is demonstrable at the abnormal angle it is usually weak, as is stereopsis. The cover test shows, of course, the typical response of a unilateral convergent squint since the fovea of the squinting eye is used for fixation if the other eye is covered.

Microtropia

This is a small-angled esotropia of less than 10^Δ in which a form of binocular single vision occurs. There is a variety of clinical findings but abnormal retinal correspondence is usual and eccentric fixation common; this may be absolute (p. 67) so that no deviation is revealed on cover test (microtropia with identity) and this fact, coupled with the excellent cosmetic appearance, makes visuscopic examination an essential diagnostic test for all patients. Patients showing microtropia without identity have central fixation or non-absolute eccentric fixation but, again, there is some form of binocular single vision, either through abnormal retinal correspondence or by way of normal retinal correspondence with central suppression and fusion of the peripheral field.

Microtropia with a latent component

This not uncommon form of microtropia may be recognised by a series of characteristic findings together forming the complete picture. (In the past an alternative name for this condition was monofixational esophoria.)

Cover test. The response to this test is unique and it requires careful performance if the diagnosis is not to be missed. The first part of the cover test is to check the bi-foveal fixation is being maintained (p. 16), and when this test is carried out it will be seen that one eye makes a fractional outward movement to take up foveal fixation, as if there were a particularly small manifest convergent squint. The movement, which is in the region of 1° or 2°, will only be seen if a close watch is kept at the moment of dissociation; an occluding card makes this easier and movement is more obvious if the examiner watches the limbus against the upper lashes. In order to check for the latent component, the eye which was seen to make the fixation movement is occluded and the cover test for heterophoria is carried out; a moderate esophoric response will be seen, the recovery often being rapid. However, if the other eye is now covered again, it will be noted that this recovery was incomplete and the final flick outwards for foveal fixation remains. This characteristic cover test of a latent convergence with a partial recovery is unilateral, occurring in the deviating eye; the other eye makes a complete recovery to foveal fixation.

Visual acuity. Very slight amblyopia in the affected eye, usually only one line less than in the normal eye, is revealed by this test. Visuscope examination is essential.

Binocular tests. Tests such as Bagolini glasses, Worth's lights and bar reading, give results consistent with the maintenance of binocular single vision although the small flick on cover test can be demonstrated while the tests are being carried out.

The four-diopter prism test. A $4^\triangle$ prism is placed base out before the supposedly fixing eye; this will result in adduction of that eye to restore foveal fixation and, by Hering's law, abduction of the other eye. The examiner watches the eye without the prism and, if binocular single vision is to be maintained, the abduction induced by Hering's law will immediately be followed by adduction as the corrective fusion reflex re-aligns the foveae to overcome diplopia. If this controlling movement does not occur the image on this minutely abducted eye must be falling on a suppression scotoma which is preventing fusion.

The eye movements induced by a prism of this power are, of course, very fine and again are best seen by watching the limbus against the upper eylashes. A $4^\triangle$ prism placed before a deviating eye will produce no eye movements at all as the displaced image still falls within the suppression scotoma and is not a disturbing factor to the foveal fixation being maintained by the other eye.

The major amblyoscope. This reveals the presence of abnormal retinal correspondence with an angle of anomaly of 1° or 2° caused by the fact that the patient uses the fovea for monocular fixation during the objective measurement of the angle and uses a parafoveal point for binocular vision during subjective testing. Fusion is usually strong and stereopsis is present.

Further tests
The investigations to date will have assessed the type of deviation by means of the cover test, the fixation, the angle of deviation and the state of binocular function. In cases where binocular single vision is present or intermittently present on the cover test, there are further tests which have to be carried out on a literate child to ascertain the circumstances under which binocular single vision is maintained; these are the investigation of binocular visual acuity and the ability to bar-read. If a deviation becomes more marked on accommodation an assessment of the AC/A ratio can be useful and in all cases, whether or not binocular single vision is being maintained, convergence should be tested.

Binocular visual acuity
Tests should be carried out at six metres and a third of a metre, using Snellens test type and reduced Snellens for near. The patient is asked to read the test type at the required distance and the cover test is

carried out to ensure that binocular single vision is being maintained. The patient should be able to maintain binocular visual acuity equal to the acuity of the weaker eye, but it is frequently found that although the cover test, when fixing a light, had shown binocular single vision, when an accommodative effort is required to read the test type a manifest deviation occurs. If this is the case, clearly the patient is squinting during his day-to-day activities at school as is either suppressing or experiencing diplopia.

Bar reading

Physiological diplopia is the basis of this test. A thumb bar reader (Plate VI) is held on the bottom of the page by the hand holding the book, and the patient is required to read continuous text while his head is held still. Either the Moorfields or the Maclure bar reading book (Plate VII) is normally used for this purpose. In order to read the full line of print it is necessary for the patient to appreciate physiological diplopia of the bar. Some patients may not actually see two bars, but state that they can 'see through the bar'. If the bar blocks out part of the page one eye only is being used. This is a finer test than simply recording the binocular visual acuity for near, as the presence of the bar may disturb a slender hold on binocular single vision. Ability to bar read small print fluently is proof of very stable binocular single vision, whereas inability indicates likelihood of decompensation.

Convergence

In the examination of squint convergence should be tested. The R.A.F. near point rule is used. In cases with binocular single vision (e.g. fully accommodative squint) binocular convergence should be 8 cm or better and well maintained; otherwise treatment is indicated as failure may cause symptoms.

In the presence of a constant deviation if binocular convergence appears to be present after the intersection of the visual axes, it should be noted. This may be the only indication of the likelihood of a functional result in a child too young to co-operate for other tests. Poor convergence or marked divergence of the deviating eye after the interesection of the visual axes is of significance in planning surgery in order to prevent the risk of consecutive divergence.

MUSCULAR ACTION

Defects of conjugate muscle action can be investigated in a variety of ways to diagnose the muscles concerned in the imbalance.

Ocular movements

These may be examined by the simple procedure of watching the patient's eyes while they are rotated into the nine cardinal positions of gaze and a thorough investigation will include movements on pursuit and command as well as 'doll's head' movements. The patient's glasses, if worn, should be removed for this test, as they obscure the examiner's view, and a pen-torch is best for fixation so that corneal reflections are created.

The examiner holds the torch straight ahead of the patient (the primary position) at about 33 cm. The directions into which the torch is now moved are those which could be described as the 'lines of the Union Jack' returning each time to the primary position between testing the successive positions since this makes any defect of movement very much more apparent. The patient follows the torch binocularly while the head, of course, remains still and the examiner observes the corneal reflections. When testing movements of depression the upper lids should be lightly restrained from their natural closing action with thumb and forefinger so that a better view of the eyes is achieved. It is often misleading to judge the symmetry of ocular movements by the relative position of the eyes against the lids because asymmetry of the palpebral fissures often gives an appearance of a defect where, in fact, perfect parallelism exists. For example, a child with epicanthus may appear to have over-acting medial recti and even an upshoot on elevation-in adduction, whereas in reality there is no defect of movement but the cornea is partially covered by the epicanthal fold.

Horizontal movements (Fig. 20). A test of *dextro version* will illustrate the action of the left medial rectus and the right lateral rectus, and *laevo version* will illustrate the action of the left lateral rectus and the right medial rectus.

Vertical movements (Fig. 20). A test of *elevation* will illustrate the combined action of the superior recti and the inferior obliques and also help in the exposure of an A or V phenomenon (see below), while *depression* will illustrate the combined action of the inferior recti and the superior obliques and again will demonstrate an A or V phenomenon.

The A and V phenomena. These are the names given, by way of graphic description, to deviations (either latent or manifest) which show a variation in their horizontal size as the fixation point moves upwards and downwards. Thus convergence increases or divergence decreases on elevation in an A phenomenon while on depression convergence decreases and divergence increases. Conversely, in a V phenomenon, divergence increases on elevation and decreases on

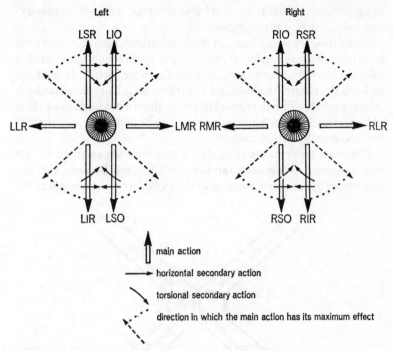

Fig. 20 Diagrammatic representation of ocular muscle actions

depression whereas convergence increases on depression and decreases on elevation.

The V phenomenon associated with convergence is characterised by an increased convergence on depression and a decreased convergence on elevation while an A phenomenon with convergence will show increased convergence on elevation and a decrease in the deviation on depression.

The V phenomenon associated with divergence is a situation in which the divergence increases on elevation and decreases on depression; divergence with an A phenomenon will show an increase of the deviation on depression and a decrease on elevation.

X and ◊ phenomena have also been recorded in which divergence (X) or convergence (◊) increases in both elevation and depression. Purely relative divergence in elevation is sometimes referred to as a Y phenomenon, relative divergence in depression as a Λ.

Cases in which binocular single vision can be maintained in the position in which the deviation is minimal, but who have a manifest squint in the opposite direction may adopt an abnormal head posture in order to achieve binocular single vision—another reason why the head position should be carefully observed and, if necessary, controlled, during investigation.

Many theories of the cause of these sometimes bizarre movements have been proposed: general consensus of opinion now suggests that bilateral inferior oblique overaction produces the V effect in both exo and eso deviations and bilateral superior oblique overactions the A effect, probably due to sagittalisation or abnormal insertion of these oblique muscles; less frequently there may be abnormal insertions of the horizontally-acting muscles.

Diagonal movements (Fig. 21). These tests are essential in that they differentiate between the two elevators and between the two depressors by requiring rotation of the globe into positions where the

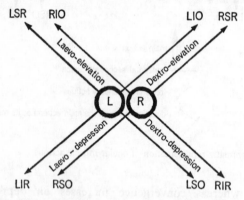

Fig. 21 Diagram illustrating 'yoke muscles' in diagonal movements

relative power of their main actions is very unequal. Thus on *dextro elevation* the right superior rectus and the left inferior oblique are tested, since the right inferior oblique and the left superior rectus have minimal elevating power in this position (although their secondary actions will now have come into play). *Laevo elevation* will test the main action of the right inferior oblique and the left superior rectus. *Laevo depression* will test the main action of the right superior oblique and the left inferior rectus. *Dextro depression* will test the main action of the right inferior rectus and the left superior oblique. The pairs of muscles involved in these movements can be referred to as 'yoke muscles'.

On binocular testing an abnormality of conjugate muscle action may be apparent either in the form of an overaction of movement of one eye, or a limitation of movement of the other, depending on which eye is actually fixing. A great variety of factors will govern this, some of the more obvious ones being, for example, that a hypotropic eye may be preferred regardless of whether the palsy is of an elevator of that eye or a depressor of the other eye; also that fixing with the paretic eye may separate the diplopia to a less tiresome position; alternatively the eye with the better visual acuity may be used for fixation—or, quite simply, on horizontal versions the nose may have 'occluded' the adducted eye.

If any asymmetry of movement is detected, a cover test in the direction of the defect will confirm its presence by requiring monocular fixation in that direction. In this way the paretic muscle will show underaction when the unaffected muscle is controlling fixation, and, when the affected eye is fixing, the excessive innervation required by the paretic muscle will cause overaction of the eye behind the cover.

Inconcomitance

A variation in the size of the deviation depending on the direction of gaze and the eye fixing is an indication of a palsy of an extrinsic ocular muscle. The inconcomitance may be apparent on cover test and on ocular movements, or it may be slight enough only to be surely demonstrated on the major amblyoscope. The actual size of the horizontal, vertical and torsional elements of a squint can be measured on this instrument fixing with either eye and in all nine cardinal positions. The larger angle is induced when fixing with the eye with the paretic muscle, and the deviation is greatest in the direction of the main action of that muscle, e.g. in case of right superior rectus palsy, the maximum deviation will be when fixing with the right eye on dextroelevation.

When measuring the deviation in the nine cardinal positions of gaze on the major amblyoscope, fixation is taken up 15° to right and left from the primary position, and elevated and depressed by 15°. This is achieved by adjusting the position of the tubes.

Mechanical restriction. If the ocular movements show atypical innervational patterns (which can be confirmed with Hess charts, as in Figure 27 or by testing the uniocular fields of fixation on the perimeter) mechanical restrictions may be suspected. Careful examination with red and green goggles will reveal atypical reversal of diplopia in extreme movements and forced duction tests and X-ray will complete the clinical picture. For instance where the inferior rectus is mechanically restricted due either to thyroid dyfunction or to tethering after a blow-out fracture, the eye will show underaction in both elevation and depression, the diplopia test revealing the image seen by the affected eye to be the higher of the two in elevation and the lower in depression.

The Hess chart

By means of whichever adaptation is preferred, this is the most excellent method of investigating the nature and extent of extra-ocular muscle imbalance. While dissociating the eyes by red and green goggles (or, in one adaptation, a mirror) the two maculae are stimulated by differing objects, the fixing eye by a spot, and the non-fixing eye by a marker. The patient is required to place the marker on the spot (Plate VIII). First one eye then the other fixes the spots in the cardinal positions of gaze. Thus Hering's law of equal innervation is utilised as a means of pin-pointing the paresis.

When using an adaptation based on colour dissociation, goggles are worn by the patient with, firstly, red before the right eye so that his right eye can see the spots on the screen before him; the left eye, however, can only see the green marker he is given to use. The red spots on the screen are now indicated to the patient in turn and, while he fixes, the innervation to the extra-ocular muscles of both eyes will be governed by that required for the right eye behind the red goggle. The patient places his green marker 'over' the red spot, i.e. he indicates the point to which the left fovea is directed, since by so doing he sees the two foveal images, the red and the green, superimposed. Plate VIII shows the old non-electrical screen, which is easier to depict, the examiner using a red-filtered torch and the patient a green one.

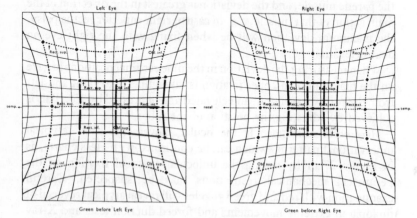

Fig. 22 Hess chart showing right lateral rectus palsy

Thus, when the red goggle is before the right eye, the movement of the left eye is being plotted while its innervation is governed by that of the right eye. If, for example, the right lateral rectus is paretic (Fig. 22) excessive innervation will be demanded by the right eye to take up fixation of the spot on the right temporal field and thus excessive innervation will be received by the left medial rectus, causing it to overact. The green marker will therefore indicate a point on the screen which is beyond the correct alignment. Alternatively, if the left medial rectus were the paretic muscle, and the right eye unaffected, only a normal stimulus would be required by the right eye to fix this spot; however, the left medial rectus, receiving only normal stimulus, and being paretic, would show an underaction, and the green marker would fall short of the correct alignment.

Having plotted on the chart the relative positions of the left eye while the right eye fixes in the cardinal positions, the goggles are now changed so that the red is before the left eye and the actions of the right eye are recorded, the innervation being governed by the left.

This test is purely subjective and can only be properly performed if the patient has normal retinal correspondence; it is not possible if he has lack of retinal correspondence since he cannot superimpose the two macular images, and it is inaccurate if he has abnormal retinal correspondence. In most cases of recently acquired palsy this is not a problem, but cases of longstanding palsy should have their binocular function assessed on the major amblyoscope before attempting a Hess chart.

Interpretation. This is made by comparing the two charts and, from what has been said, it will be seen that the more restricted chart will be that of the eye with the paretic muscle, the other chart being enlarged by the inevitable overaction. In particular the smaller field will show its greatest restriction in the direction of the main action of the paretic muscle, and since these are clearly labelled on the charts there should be no difficulty in diagnosis! It is important not to mistake displacement for restriction or enlargement. If the individual squares plotted by the patient are the correct size, but the position of the charts is displaced sideways, the cause is not a muscle palsy but a concomitant deviation.

The muscle sequelae will also be apparent on the chart. A very recently acquired palsy will show only the primary paresis and the dramatic overaction of the contralateral synergist (Fig. 23). The fields are very inconcomitant and diagnosis is simple. As the secondary contracture and limitation occur, the shape of the chart changes (Fig. 24). Both eyes now show restricted action in one direction; the primarily paresed muscle is, of course, still weak, but its contralateral antagonist is also noticeably restricted in its movement. There is also an overaction in both eyes: the original overaction (that of the contralateral synergist to the primarily paresed muscle) remains in a rather reduced intensity, but the ipsilateral antagonist is also showing

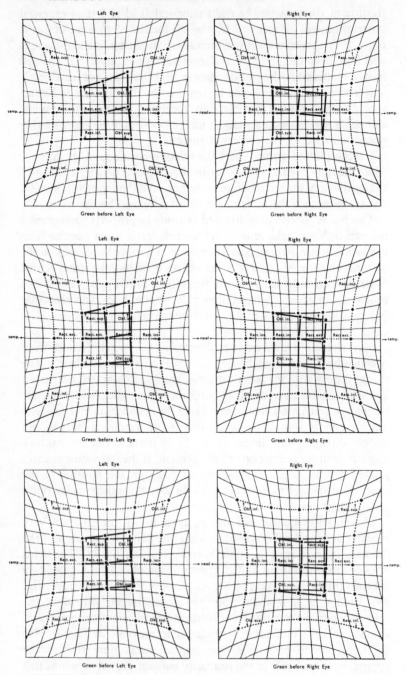

Figs 23, 24, 25 The development of concomitance

overaction. Thus the two fields become gradually more and more concomitant with the passage of time until it may become quite difficult to determine which was the primarily paretic muscle (Fig. 25).

In this event it is useful to remember that if the two fields are very concomitant and the two limitations of action seen in a pair of contralateral antagonists are so similar as to make the diagnosis obscure, the overactions may be more revealing. The overaction of the contralateral synergist to the primarily paretic muscle usually remains very slightly greater than that of the ipsilateral antagonist. Thus in Figure 25 the right superior rectus and the left superior oblique show identical limitation, but the overaction of the left inferior oblique is slightly greater than that of the right inferior rectus, indicating that the limited muscle which suffered the primary paresis was, in fact, the right superior rectus.

When the defect is obvious it may be identified from the inner 'square' alone but a very slight imbalance may only become evident on extreme movement and therefore be virtually undetected on the inner field (Fig. 26). The relative shape of the inner and outer fields is also

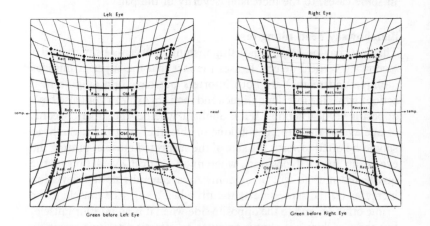

Fig. 26 Hess chart demonstrating innervational defect

significant, the 'squares' being definitely asymmetrically distorted in an innervational defect, but tending to remain unchanged or more symmetrical in a mechanical defect—compare Figures 26 and 27. That is to say that a mechanical restriction is the exception to the guiding pattern; in Figure 27 there is restriction of the left inferior rectus after a blow-out fracture: the left eye is tethered and limited in elevation and depression, the right eye showing compensatory overaction straight up and down. If there were also an innervational

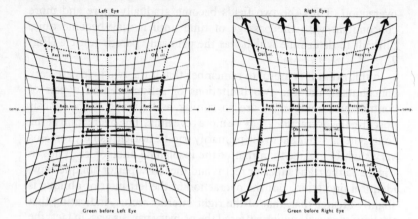

Fig. 27 Hess chart demonstrating mechanical restriction

defect of a left elevator there would be overactions of the contralateral synergist(s) but these normal muscle sequelae are plainly absent.

Hess charts have their value not only in the original diagnosis of the paresis, but also as a guide to the progress of spontaneous recovery or, in some cases, to the increasing severity of the palsy.

Bielchowsky head tilting test

This test may be helpful in distinguishing between a primary and a secondary vertical defect. It uses the fact that the superior muscles (oblique and rectus) are both intorters but have opposing vertical actions while the inferior obliques and recti are extorters but also have opposing vertical actions. If it is doubtful whether the superior rectus of one eye or the superior oblique of the other is at fault, the head should be tilted towards the side of the suspected muscle, putting the eye in an intorted position, whereupon vertical overaction of the unaffected muscle will be evident. As a general rule the deviation increases on the same side as the tilt when a superior muscle is the prime offender and to the opposite side when it is an inferior muscle, but the test does not always produce an effective positive result.

POSTURAL DEFECTS

To investigate an abnormal head posture it is best to have made no comment about it beforehand because once the patient is conscious that his posture is under consideration it is almost impossible for him to retain his customary position. It is best if a child is standing, and an adult should certainly not be reviewed while sitting sideways in a chair. In every case the examiner faces the patient squarely.

The turn is most easily seen by comparing the perspective of the two temples, and spectacles make this easier still. The tilt is best considered by deciding if the nasal bone is vertical, or again, spectacle frames give a very useful line. The chin elevation is the most difficult to assess if it is not marked and possibly a profile view is the best one.

Having assessed the abnormal head posture the cover test should be done with the head in this position. The examiner should then straighten the head without comment and repeat the cover test for comparison. It can then be seen if the head returns to the abnormal position when the patient relaxes again after the cover test and only now should the question of the head posture be discussed.

To record an abnormal head posture a photograph is ideal, but a description or a sketch diagram will do. If the patient has old photographs of childhood the duration of the muscle palsy can sometimes be very strikingly proved.

Finally, in warning, it should be repeated that many cases do not show the abnormal head posture which entirely conforms to the theoretical position which should compensate for the palsy concerned. It is therefore extremely unwise to attempt any kind of diagnosis of muscle palsy solely from the head posture which has been adopted.

Ocular torticollis

The ocular torticollis should be easily distinguished from non-ocular torticollis because the abnormal head posture may be in any of the possible combinations of the three component parts. But even if it is similar to that of the orthopaedic torticollis (with the chin up, the head tilt to one shoulder and turned to the opposite side) the differential diagnosis is clear because the patient can voluntarily straighten the head and also usually has unrestricted movement in all directions. Added to this an imbalance will be seen on testing ocular movements and the cover test will reveal a vertical squint. If the ocular torticollis completely compensates the muscular imbalance the deviation will not be manifest when the patient holds his head in his customary way, but will be manifest when the head is straight. It is possible, however, that the deviation is no longer compensated by the head posture and a manifest squint may be present all the time, increasing when the head is straight.

ANOMALOUS FINDINGS

There is, of course, a variety of anomalies which may be found during the investigation; some of the more common are dealt with on page

153 where surgical procedures are considered, but in addition the following may be noted.

Marcus Gunn (jaw-winking) phenomenon. There is unilateral ptosis which increases if the jaw is deviated to the same side, but the lid retracts if the mouth is opened or the jaw deviated to the other side.

Aberrant third nerve (misdirection syndrome). Incorrect regeneration of nerve fibres after injury results in partial ptosis and bizarre ocular movements. The levator receives innervation intended for the inferior rectus causing retraction of the lid on depression of the eye (pseudo Graefe's sign); the medial rectus may also receive innervation intended for the superior rectus, causing elevation of the eye on attempted adduction and other variations have been reported.

Moebius syndrome. There is congenital bilateral paralysis of the sixth nerve associated with seventh (facial) paralysis.

Strabismus fixus. A short fibrous medial rectus attached to the globe at the equator causes the eye to be fixed in the adducted position and retracted.

GENERAL PROCEDURE

All cases will be refracted and have an ophthalmoscopic examination.

The case history will be the first part of the investigation, when particular stress should be laid on the age of onset, the possible cause and whether the squint is constant or if intermittent binocular single vision persists—or did persist for a period after onset. Any *previous treatment* should be noted, relevant *family history* and the presence of any *symptoms* should be recorded and an *abnormal head posture*, if present, will be observed during this questioning.

The cover test should follow since *the visual acuity* is sometimes better investigated after the cover test so that the possibly-amblyopic eye is checked first; it is extraordinary how many patients will recite the first few letters from memory rather than reveal gross amblyopia. *Binocular visual acuity* should be tested at 6 metres and a third of a metre, followed by *bar-reading*.

Ocular movements should next be investigated with a torch but in cases with obvious limitations of movement the surgeon may require a *forced duction test* (that is, mechanical movement of the eyes in all directions of gaze under local or general anaesthetic, depending on the age of the patient). This will indicate whether the defect is a weakness of a muscle or a mechanical obstruction. *Convergence*, either binocular or in the presence of a manifest deviation, should be measured. *Diplopia tests* are carried out and, if there is inconcomitance, a note should be made of the direction in which the images are most widely separated. The relative position of the two images, and which eyes sees the further image, should also be recorded.

Measurement of the deviation will now be assessed by means of:
Prism cover test, for comparison of near and distant deviation.
Major amblyoscope—fixing either eye in all directions of gaze.
By corneal reflections in infants, and cases of eccentric fixation.

Investigation of binocular function on the major amblyoscope starts with an assessment of whether or not normal retinal correspondence is present.

1. If normal retinal correspondence is present (a) investigate whether fusion power remains, and its potential strength; (b) test for stereopsis.
2. If normal retinal correspondence has been lost (a) investigate area of suppression; (b) test for abnormal retinal correspondence.

Any other specialised tests are used where appropriate such as Hess charts, fields of binocular single vision, Bagolini glasses, Worth lights, Bielchowsky after-image test, past pointing and tests for the risk of post-operative diplopia.

Clinical photography can play a useful part as a record of ocular movements and of head posture at a given time. Childhood snaps can also illustrate dramatically the age of onset, either by revealing the squint itself or the adoption of a head posture.

Because it may create an after-image which prohibits further tests, the *visuscope* investigation must be left till the end of any investigation session. Examination should be carried out on all patients with 6/12 vision or less in the amblyopic eye.

Investigation of an infant

The general procedure must, of course, be modified when the patient is very young. A friendly non-clinical atmosphere with toys and pictures is important and experience with small children is an asset. *Ocular movements* in nine positions of gaze may well be achieved during preliminary overtures, either by moving an attractive squeaking toy or possibly by shifting the child bodily into relative positions. *Head posture* or facial asymmetry should be carefully observed meanwhile.

The *distance cover test* is sometimes obtainable with the help of an assistant attracting attention with the same squeaking toy at the other side of the room. The *near cover test* is carried out with a winking torch to capture the child's interest and so that the reflections can be observed. Ocular movements are now confirmed.

The *state of fixation* should be assessed carefully. If the child is very restless a plaster occlusion may have to be put for a few moments over each eye in turn while watching how steadily he can fix the light, but violent resistance to having the normally fixing eye covered may be the only evidence forthcoming that the other eye has reduced visual acuity. This *visual acuity* can be further checked by using simple optokinetic apparatus, by the Catford drum or by rolling small balls of graded size. Most infants also need little encouragement to pick up tiny edible balls such as 'hundreds and thousands'. For detailed comments on testing visual acuity of infant patients, see page 63.

It may be possible to *measure the deviation* by prism reflection test but many infants turn their head away when the prism bar is put close to their eyes, so Hirschberg's reflections may have to be used, as the major amblyoscope is usually unsuitable for any under about 2 years old.

Examination with the *visuscope* will confirm the point of fixation, the extent of amblyopia being relative to the distance of an eccentric point from the fovea; this test is carried out last because of the after image it induces.

If there is any suspicion of a bilateral external rectus palsy, an *occlusion test* should be carried out between visits to confirm or refute it. Not infrequently a patient with alternating convergent squint adopts the tripartite field of fixation (using the convergent right eye for fixation in the left field and the convergent left eye for fixation in the right field) and consequently never requires the full use of the lateral recti. A mild paresis becomes, therefore, a marked limitation due to habitual disuse, and a simple test of ocular movements, even if examined monocularly, will not be sufficient to induce their action. A brief period of total occlusion should be carried out. This must not be more than 5 to 10 minutes for an infant within the sensitive period, but should be up to 3 or 4 days for an older child, after which the abducting power of the unoccluded eye may be reviewed. The test is then repeated for the other eye and by this means the amount of surgery considered necessary to correct the deviation may be planned more soundly.

A confident report may only be possible after several visits—particularly if no abnormality is detected but it is most important to reach a confident conclusion in infant cases. Sufficient evidence can be gathered as early as 6 months of age to enable useful preventive and/or corrective treatment to be started. Early detection of any obstacles to binocular function may be vital to normal development of fusion and stereopsis, while secondary complications of amblyopia and abnormal retinal correspondence can be averted.

The qualified orthoptist is trained to carry out all the investigations described in this chapter, with the exception of the ophthalmoscopy, photography and forced duction test.

9

Factors influencing prognosis

The wise selection of cases for treatment is possibly one of the most important features of good medical care and therefore a thorough grasp of the factors which influence the prognosis in cases of squint is quite essential. However before considering these factors it is important to appreciate the criteria by which a case of squint may be discharged as orthoptically satisfactory.

STANDARD FOR DISCHARGE

In order to reach this standard the patient, with any refractive error corrected, should have the ability to maintain comfortable binocular single vision for all distances and in all directions of gaze without the adoption of an abnormal head posture. This binocular single vision must be entirely symptom-free. If hypermetropia is present, binocular single vision should be maintained even when correction of the manifest hypermetropia is reduced by three dioptre spheres. Certain tests are of special significance in confirming that the standard has been reached.

On cover test there should be a rapid recovery to binocular single vision on removal of the cover.

With any refractive error corrected the binocular visual acuity for near and distance should be as good as that of the eye with the lower visual acuity, and the patient should have the ability to bar-read N.5 or print of a size read by the weaker eye. Where hypermetropia is present, binocular visual acuity and bar-reading of the same standard as that achieved while the glasses are worn should be maintained when the correction of the manifest hypermetropia is reduced by 3 DS.

The near point of convergence should be 8 cm or better, and should be well-maintained.

This, then, is the standard which is the goal in treatment of squint, and so, in assessing the prognosis and in planning the treatment, this goal should be kept constantly in mind.

Unfortunately there are all too many patients who do not reach this standard—they may only achieve binocular single vision intermittently, or, through lack of binocular function, they have to be content with an adequate cosmetic appearance. In these cases the aim before discharge is to achieve and maintain as good a visual acuity as possible in the amblyopic eye without subjecting the patient to insuperable diplopia.

There are therefore two aspects of treatment to be considered: treatment of any amblyopia to restore good visual acuity, and treatment of the actual squint. Since the defects, the aim of the treatment and the treatment itself are completely different for the two conditions, they are considered separately and Chapter 7 is devoted exclusively to problems of visual acuity.

The prognosis in manifest squint is a very intricate matter of the interplay of factors and, for the sake of clarity, these would seem best considered in four major groups.

GROUP A

This group contains the factors which might be regarded as those principally influencing the prognosis.

Occasional binocular single vision in an intermittent squint is a strong factor in favour of a good prognosis.

The present age of the patient is of great importance, particularly in a constant squint. When it is remembered that the conditioned binocular reflexes develop within the first few years of life it will be appreciated that the period of time during which the restoration of parallel visual axes can result in binocular single vision is also very limited. It is a reasonable generalisation to say that the younger the patient is when treatment is undertaken the better is its chance of success. This statement, however, is intricately influenced by the other aspects of the prognosis yet to be considered.

The binocular function potentially available in the case of a manifest squint must be known before a sure prognosis can be made; this is diagnosed on the major amblyoscope and with the prism bar.

If all grades of binocular vision are present the prognosis is greatly enhanced. This factor would, therefore, make the child's age much less significant and even if the fusional reserve is somewhat weakened, it is often possible to strengthen it by orthoptic exercises.

If there is no fusion, in that the reserve is negligible although the patient can demonstrate normal retinal correspondence, the prognosis is considerably less good and the age factor becomes very much more important. If the orthoptist is of the opinion that the remnants of fusion were masked by suppression on the major amblyoscope and if the patient is only 3 or 4 years old a short course of treatment might be desirable to support the diagnosis. The absence of fusion, once confirmed, is an insurmountable factor against a good prognosis.

If there is lack of retinal correspondence there can, of course, be no fusion. However it is possible again that the orthoptist may consider the major amblyoscope findings to have been exaggerated by a dense central suppression area and a 3 or 4 year old patient might benefit from a short course of treatment to verify the true situation.

If there is abnormal retinal correspondence the prognosis for normal binocular single vision is almost certainly poor because abnormal retinal correspondence is very difficult to eliminate. But for patients with microtropia and in other instances in which the appearance is acceptable, abnormal retinal correspondence is a useful deterrant to the recurrence of amblyopia and to the development of consecutive divergence—at the same time providing the patient with a form of binocular vision—and so it should be encouraged.

The influence of the major amblyoscope findings on the prognosis is inevitably very strong indeed but, coupled with the written record of these tests, the opinion of the examiner who carried out the investigation should also be considered. Wide experience in handling the major amblyoscope is invaluable in enabling the examiner to differentiate between the infinite shades of degree to which the degeneration of normal binocular function may have progressed.

There is however a large group of children under the age of three and sometimes older, in which it is impossible accurately to assess the state of binocular function due to difficulty in getting reliable subjective responses to tests. Certain tests, such as the patient's ability to maintain binocular convergence after the crossing of the visual axes, may indicate the presence of binocular function. Inability to elicit binocular function in young children is no reason to delay treatment if other factors such as occasional binocular single vision, the present age, the age of onset or a short duration of squint suggest the possibility of a good prognosis.

The age of onset must also find a place in this group but, although a prognostic factor of great theoretical importance, it is in practical terms frequently overshadowed by the two giants already discussed. The age of onset indicates the stage which reflex development had reached prior to their interruption by the squint (but in practice there is frequently no clear knowledge of exactly when the squint did first appear). A definite history of congenital onset is a factor against a really good prognosis since the conditioned reflexes will not have developed at all; on the other hand, if the child is still under 2, so that much of the period for reflex development remains, speedy surgery may establish binocular single vision. Almost without exception the full significance of the age of onset is only apparent when coupled with the present age (i.e. the age when first seen by an ophthalmologist).

The duration of the squint, this is, the time lag between the age of onset and the present age, is, in effect, almost more important than the age of onset. Thus a congenital squint may yet develop binocular single vision with very early surgery so that the squinting period is short. The interpretation of the major amblyoscope findings may also be influenced by this factor—for instance, suppression and gross amblyopia can develop with amazing rapidity in children with an onset of squint at three years of age, and a history of short duration could be a factor encouraging treatment in spite of an apparently unsatisfactory binocular state.

GROUP B

This comprises factors which can be just as significant towards the formation of a prognosis as those in Group A, but they are not an inevitable aspect of all cases, as are the factors already discussed.

A *unilateral visual defect* which results in a significant difference in the clarity of the two images is an obvious barrier to the maintenance of binocular single vision.

Amblyopia which has failed to respond to treatment is, then, a factor against a good prognosis since a sharp image and an unclear one are not easy to fuse.

Anisometropia can have the same effect and may also, in marked cases, result in aniseikonia, which makes fusion impossible if it is other than slight.

An opacity of the media or any other interruption to normal retinal sensation may also disrupt binocular co-ordination.

Nystagmus is another factor which, if present, reduces the likelihood of restoring binocular single vision. Manifest nystagmus (that is, one which is constantly present) is a permanent disturbance of visual function and prevents any kind of treatment other than surgery. Latent nystagmus (one which only occurs on dissocation) reduces the visual acuity of the unoccluded eye and may hamper treatment.

Previous treatment should be noted for the same reason as in the case of amblyopia: the prognosis is better the sooner treatment is begun and if it has failed in the past, after a shorter duration of squint, it is not likely to succeed after a longer one. This fact should, however, be considered in conjunction with the co-operation the patient would be able to contribute at the two periods in question.

GROUP C

This may be regarded as a group of factors whose influence on the prognosis is in the nature of a complication, for in the presence of these circumstances the treatment is much less straightforward. Thus even if the other factors in the case suggest a good prognosis a completely satisfactory state on discharge may not be achieved.

Inconcomitance is a factor which almost inevitably prevents the maintenance of binocular single vision in all positions of gaze, for if the angle of squint varies in different directions it is not likely to be controlled throughout the variations. Pre-operative orthoptic treatment in cases with inconcomitance is virtually impossible because the adjustment of the major amblyoscope tubes which is correct in one position will not result in bi-foveal stimulation in another so that suppression may be very difficult to overcome and fusion almost impossible to exercise. If the inconcomitant squint has its onset in adult life the prognosis for binocular single vision is far better than for a child as orthoptic treatment is rarely necessary.

Surgical treatment requires careful planning and it is very possible that a series of operations may be necessary before a perfect result is achieved.

A small angle of squint also has an adverse influence on prognosis. A horizontal deviation of less than 5° is very difficult to eradicate. It is not uncommon to see cases with deviations of this size and with dense central suppression but all grades of binocular vision demonstrable on the synoptophore—and yet there is poor response to all attempts to teach control of the angle by orthoptic methods and even quite liberal surgery results in the same manifest deviation persisting. Occlusion to ensure maximum visual acuity and treatment to strengthen this gross fusion is all that is required.

A vertical deviation of less than 4^Δ is also troublesome. The normal vertical fusional reserve is very small indeed (averaging 3^Δ or 4^Δ) and so even the smallest of vertical elements may be sufficient to prevent the patient from overcoming a basically horizontal deviation which could otherwise be controlled. These very tiny vertical deviations are frequently not desirable targets for surgery but may in fact respond well to the prescription of a vertical prism.

The co-operation a patient is able to give to treatment is of great importance. Only a very limited amount of orthoptic treatment can be given without active participation by the patient and this may be inadequate either because the child is too lethargic or inarticulate to respond intelligently to the constant questioning and discussion which is an essential part of orthoptic treatment, or because he is too alert or impetuous to concentrate for more than a moment at a time. Co-operation from the parents must also be forthcoming both in the matter of arranging for frequent attendance and also in supervising homework exercises.

It must be acknowledged that the willingness of patient and parent to co-operate will be the direct result of the interest shown by the ophthalmologist and the patience exerted by the orthoptist; ability to co-operate then remains the only hazard.

GROUP D

The general considerations which are occasionally involved when treatment is necessary from this group.

General health can be a disrupting factor, particularly if frequent or chronic illness prevents regular attendance or if some general condition prohibits surgery.

The economic factor is another which can influence the prognosis; if both parents are working weekly attendance may be an arrangement they are not able to make or there may be a variety of other personal problems which, even in a welfare state, stand in the way of an otherwise good prognosis. Squint treatment is so much a matter which is complicated by delay that to postpone it until domestic circumstances are easier may mean the difference between success and failure.

Family history of squint is a depressing factor in the prognosis but not one which should be allowed to sway the selection for treatment.

SUMMARY

It might be appropriate to quote the titles one has given to the four groups of prognostic factors when teaching orthoptic students; these are hardly offered as a serious classification, but have been found a help in learning the art of prognosis.

Group A are absolute essentials, always to be considered.

Group B are brickwalls if found to be present.

Group C are complications demanding great skill if they are to be overcome.

Group D are difficulties of a non-ophthalmic nature which may need to be considered.

It should be said here that not only does preventive treatment following early detection give a better prognosis for binocular function, but it also avoids years of tedious corrective measures for secondary complications later. It cannot be too strongly emphasised that the best prognosis in cases of constant childhood squint is in those cases receiving early therapy.

THE ROLE OF THE ORTHOPTIST

The orthoptist's opinion is important in the formation of the prognosis since the interpretation of so many findings is coloured by the indefinable implications of the patient's technique in performing the tests. The orthoptist has also had an opportunity of forming an opinion of the co-operation to be expected and she is trained to be aware of the relative significance of the diagnostic features of the case.

10

Classification

While it is acknowledged that rigid classification is never strictly possible, it is also granted that many squints fall into particular groups and it is of value, therefore, to define the classic conditions which occur.

PSEUDO-SQUINT

There is a variety of factors which can lead to the appearance of a squint where, in fact, no squint is present and constant binocular single vision is being maintained. In these cases it is plainly most important to be entirely certain that the appearance is deceptive and no true squint exists before the patient is discharged. This can satisfactorily be done by a conclusive cover test and by the demonstration of phenomena only associated with binocular single vision, such as the appreciation of stereopsis and the ability to overcome a base out prism and, on its removal, to take up bifoveal fixation again. In the case of young children, discharge should be delayed until accurate visual acuity is obtained and the child is able to demonstrate binocular function subjectively. This is particularly important where there is a family history of squint. It is not unknown for a child to attend several times exhibiting a latent deviation before a 'true squint' is noted, so early discharge in these cases is inadvisable.

Facial asymmetry. A pseudo-squint of any variety may be caused by asymmetrical features, the appearance depending on the deformity concerned.

Pseudo-convergence. A convergent appearance may arise from several causes.

Epicanthus is the most common cause of pseudo-convergence. It is a condition in which there is a fold of skin over the inner canthus (which gradually lessens as the nasal bones develop). Thus the position of the cornea is apparently displaced nasally and a convergent squint is suspected, being apparently more marked on side versions as the adducted eye 'disappears' under the epicanthal fold. Asymmetrical epicanthus increases the appearance of convergent squint.

Negative angle alpha (gamma or kappa) also gives a convergent appearance (Fig. 28). Angles alpha, gamma and kappa are caused by virtue of the fact that the macula does not lie centrally at the back of

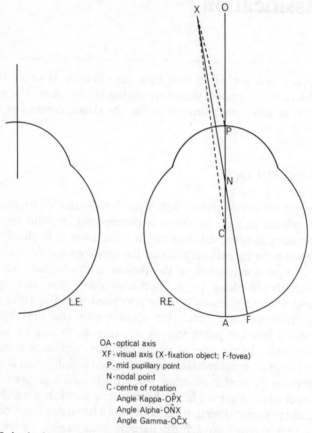

OA - optical axis
XF - visual axis (X - fixation object; F - fovea)
P - mid pupillary point
N - nodal point
C - centre of rotation
Angle Kappa - OP̂X
Angle Alpha - ON̂X
Angle Gamma - OĈX

Fig. 28 Angles kappa, alpha and gamma

the eye, but rather is slightly temporal. Thus the axis from the fovea to the fixation object normally lies at an angle of approximately 4° to the optical axis. This accounts for the slightly nasal position of the normal corneal reflection. If the fovea is temporally placed the angle alpha is termed positive, but if, unusually, the fovea is nasal, the angle is termed negative. The relative size of angles, alpha, gamma and kappa is virtually the same.

Narrow interpupillary distance and enophthalmos may also cause pseudo-convergence.

Pseudo-divergence. This may be caused by exophthalmos, wide interpupillary distance, enlarged positive angle alpha as noted above, and by heterochromia (the less dark eye appearing to be divergent).

Pseudo-hypertropia. This may be the result of unilateral ptosis.

Pseudo-hypotropia. Unilateral coloboma may produce this affect.

It should also be noted that the conditions mentioned above may mask a squint which is actually present. Thus a slight convergent squint may go unnoticed in a patient with a positive angle alpha which is larger than is normal.

MANIFEST SQUINT

The majority of cases of squint are horizontal in nature although a high proportion have both horizontal and vertical elements in the deviation. Purely vertical squints are rare and this is accounted for by the fact that the vertically acting muscles have a secondary horizontal and torsional action as well as a primary vertical one; consequently any defect in their action will have a complex effect on the ocular posture.

CONCOMITANT SQUINT

Concomitant squint is necessarily non-paretic in origin and this section, therefore, deals entirely with horizontal deviations within which there are two broad divisions—the non-accommodative squints and the accommodative squints.

Non-accommodative squints

These are unaffected by the exertion of accommodation and thus the size of the deviation is also not materially altered by the correction of any refractive error.

Accommodative squints

Such squints are influenced by the exertion of accommodation and therefore the size of the squint is significantly altered by taking up fixation of a near object or by correcting the refractive error.

A *myopic correction* will reduce a divergent deviation or increase a convergent one; cases have been seen in which binocular single vision is maintained while wearing a myopic correction, but a manifest divergent squint occurs when the glasses are removed.

A *hypermetropic correction* will reduce a convergent squint or increase a divergent one, and there will also be an increase of a convergent deviation when a near fixation object is viewed.

Table I Concomitant squint

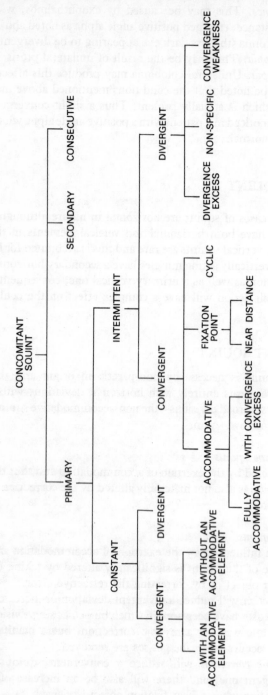

Constant squints
The majority of cases in this category are convergent, but all constant squints, regardless of direction, will of course lead to degeneration of binocular function.

Constant convergent squints
Convergent squint with an accommodative element. In this condition a manifest convergent squint is present without glasses and is substantially reduced, but not eradicated, by the wearing of a hypermetropic correction. (These cases are sometimes referred to as partially accommodative squints.) These constant squints are normally unilateral and result in the typical secondary defects associated with such a condition, i.e. amblyopia may be marked, the fusion power will continue to degenerate throughout the duration of the squint and abnormal retinal correspondence may develop. Treatment including re-assessment of the refractive error, is therefore urgent if normal binocular function is to be restored.

Convergent squints without an accommodative element. These may be unilateral or alternating: if alternating, the squint will not cause amblyopia. There is a small group of constant convergent squint with divergence weakness, i.e. the deviation increases on distant fixation.

Constant divergent squints
Constant divergent squints will have the same characteristics as those for constant convergent squints, i.e. if unilateral, amblyopia will develop, and in all cases there will be loss of binocular function throughout the squinting period.

Because the presence of a constant squint undermines binocular function, treatment should be undertaken as soon as possible if binocular single vision is to be restored.

Intermittent squints
Unlike the situation in constant squints, these patients are not suffering a perpetual suspension of binocular function and therefore the presence of the squint is not as inevitably destructive.

Intermittent convergent squints
These form the largest section of the intermittent squints and by far the greater number of the intermittent convergent squints show the characteristics of the accommodative type of deviation.
Fully accommodative convergent squint. This is a condition in which binocular single vision is constantly maintained while the

hypermetropic correction is worn, but a manifest convergent squint occurs when the glasses are removed. Amblyopia is mild and fusion is usually strong. As long as glasses are constantly worn reflex development is properly continued, and treatment to teach control of the deviation without glasses can safely be postponed until there is good co-operation.

Accommodative squint with convergence excess. In this condition binocular single vision is maintained only for distance while the hypermetropic correction is worn, a manifest convergent squint occurring for near in spite of the glasses. (There is also a small group of cases who show binocular single vision for distance and a manifest convergent squint for near although no refractive error is present.) Although, of course, the maintenance of binocular single vision for distance illustrates that fusion is still being used, these patients show moderate amblyopia and reduced fusional reserve, and treatment is not so wisely delayed as in the fully accommodative cases.

Relating to fixation distance. Although not accommodative in nature, these patients will show a manifest deviation which occurs only on attempting either near or distance fixation; these are not common and more usually are associated with a decompensating heterophoria.

Relating to time. This rare category is the cyclic squint, occuring at regular intervals as in the alternate day squint (p. 155).

Intermittent divergent squint

Such squints are not infrequently seen; they are not accommodative but relate to the fixation distance. Although fusion is not lost in intermittent squints, the divergent variety tend to show very dense suppression when squinting, preventing the recognition of pathological diplopia.

Intermittent divergent squint with divergent excess. A condition in which the patient maintains binocular single vision for near but for distance there is usually a manifest divergent squint, and there is certainly a manifest divergent squint for far distance (which is only demonstrable by carrying out the cover test using a fixation object beyond approximately 20 metres). Because it is the near position rather than the distance one which is most frequently used in everyday life, this type of squint has a particularly slow degenerative effect on binocular function.

Intermittent divergent squint with convergence weakness (in which the manifest divergent squint occurs in the near position and binocular single vision is maintained for distance). These are found most usually among adolescents associated with a decompensating exophoria. If the condition occurs in young children it will have a far more rapid effect on binocular function than the divergence excess type, since the squint is present during close work, which is the most commonly used position.

Intermittent divergent squint, non-specific type. One in which the manifest squint occurs at any distance or any time. It is not, therefore, easy to generalise on its effect on binocular function though, of course, the fact that fusion power has survived is proved by the fact that the squint remains intermittent.

By definition an intermittent squint is not constantly undermining binocular function and therefore immediate treatment may not be necessary. If periodic observation reveals that the deviation is becoming manifest more frequently, treatment becomes urgent.

Primary squint
All the types of squint already defined—constant and intermittent—are primary deviations: that is to say the deviation constitutes the initial defect, in contrast to the situation in secondary and consecutive squints.

Secondary squints
This group comprises squints which are the result of some other pathological ocular defect. For example, a secondary divergent squint is a common result of blindness.

Consecutive squints
These are deviations which have replaced a squint of the contrasting direction—thus a consecutive divergent squint is one which follows the presence of a convergent one. Consecutive convergence or divergence may occur as a result of surgery; alternatively, consecutive divergence is the natural sequence of events in a squint of long standing with no binocular function. This is because of the tendency for gradually increasing divergence of the visual axes throughout life. If the consecutive deviation is due to over-liberal surgery and fusion potential is present, there should be no delay in further treatment.

INCONCOMITANT SQUINT

Horizontal inconcomitant squint
Horizontal inconcomitant squints may be either congenital or acquired. The latter are confined almost entirely to palsies of the lateral rectus—apart from III nerve conditions. Congenital conditions may be due to either a muscle palsy (again the lateral rectus being the more commonly affected) or a musculo-fascial anomaly, and may be

Table II Inconcomitant squint

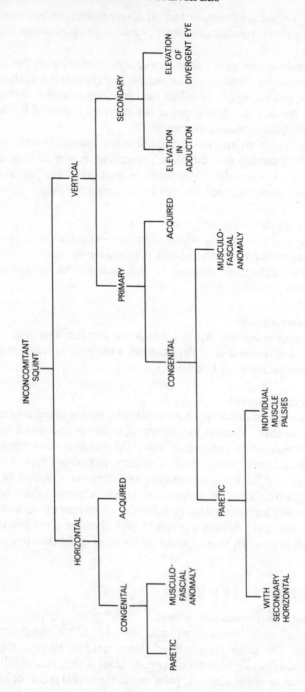

compensated by the adoption of a face turn in which case binocular function will have developed. If the palsy has resulted in a constant manifest deviation, amblyopia and loss of binocular function will occur. In either case early surgery is essential if comfortable binocular single vision is to be established. Duane's retraction syndrome is a special case; see page 154.

Vertical inconcomitant squints
Vertical inconcomitant squints are best considered as being either primary or secondary.

Primary vertical squints
A defect of one or more of the vertically acting muscles produces a primary vertical squint. The defect may be congenital or acquired.

Congenital vertical deviations. These will be due either to a muscle palsy or to a musculo-fascial anomaly.

Paretic squints. Patients in this category fall into two main groups.

1. Those with *an individual muscle palsy* showing only the typical secondary horizontal deviation. This is the type of case with which ocular torticollis may be associated. In certain cases this abnormal head posture may no longer compensate for the deviation and in others it may never have been adopted. This variation, coupled with the fact that these cases may present as infants, children or adults, means that the prognosis of any one case has to be assessed on its own merits.

2. Those with a *secondary horizontal deviation* which is significant and can be associated with hypermetropia. These patients may or may not demonstrate binocular function depending on the time of onset of the constant deviation. The prognosis is once again very variable.

Musculo-fascial anomalies. A primary vertical squint may arise from such anomalies affecting the vertically acting muscles; one example of such a condition is the superior oblique tendon sheath syndrome. The prognosis will depend on whether an abnormal head posture has been adopted and on the binocular functions.

Acquired vertical deviations. A palsy of one or more of the vertically acting muscles will give rise to an acquired vertical squint and the resultant clinical picture will vary according to the muscle or muscles affected, the severity of the palsy and the period of time which has elapsed since the palsy was acquired. The ultimate prognosis in these cases must necessarily depend on the cause of the acquired muscle palsy and if it is due to general disease the ocular prognosis may not be able to be assessed until treatment of the general condition is completed.

Secondary vertical squints

Such squints occur as a result of the presence of a horizontal manifest deviation and they may be differentiated from primary vertical squints by several factors. The horizontal element in the deviation is the major one, the vertical element being very much less apparent, and there is rarely an abnormal head posture. Neither is there a limitation of action of a vertically acting muscle—an exuberance of action may be seen, but this is not associated with any underaction of a yoke muscle.

Elevation in adduction. This is the most common form of secondary vertical squint. It becomes apparent when the gaze is directed to the side; while the abducted eye fixes the adducted one is seen to elevate. If this exuberance of the inferior oblique is not a result of a limitation of either the contralateral superior rectus or the ipsilateral superior oblique, it is plainly not paretic in origin but is secondary to the convergent squint. Chavasse explains this by the fact that in adduction the inferior oblique is at a mechanical advantage over the superior oblique. This is understood when one remembers that the inferior oblique lies at 50° to the visual axis compared with the 55° of the superior oblique and also that it is longer than the effective part of the superior oblique.

Elevation in adduction may become so habitual in a case of longstanding marked convergent squint that a small vertical element is permanently associated with the horizontal deviation.

Elevation of a divergent eye. This is also not uncommon and is seen particularly in cases of intermittent divergent squint. It is accounted for by the physiological tendency for the eyes to elevate in the divergent position.

11

Principles for the management of squint

This chapter deals with the principles governing the care of cases of squint and fuller details of the techniques employed in the various stages of treatment will be described in the suceeding two chapters. Since a unilateral visual defect can be a very strong factor against a good prognosis for manifest squint, it follows that the management of amblyopia and the management of squint may well be two sides of the same coin. Problems of visual acuity and amblyopia are considered in detail in Chapter 7.

NON-PARETIC SQUINTS

The majority of the cases seen fall into this non-paretic category. Their management will differ as widely as their individual characteristics but can be usefully considered according to their prognosis.

Cases of good prognosis

One cannot with certainty say that the prognosis is good unless it is possible to demonstrate the presence of fusion. Into this category fall cases who have intermittent binocular single vision or can demonstrate fusion potential in the presence of a constant squint.

Visual acuity

The correction of any significant refractive error is of great importance. Not only will this ensure that the retinal images are clear, which is a pre-requisite for strong fusion, but, if the refractive error has been instrumental in causing the squint, its correction may restore binocular single vision. Equally the eradication of any amblyopia is important since amblyopia is a barrier to the efficient maintenance of binocular single vision.

Orthoptic treatment for binocular function

The next stage in the management is to overcome any suppression and to ensure strong fusion with good reserves and easy stereopsis. This is accompanied by treatment to teach the recognition of pathological diplopia so that the patient is aware of the presence of the squint and so that, when binocular single vision is restored, proper subjective co-operation can be achieved by the patient in 'joining the diplopia'.

Constant squints. This treatment should be carried out as early as possible so that the restoration of binocular single vision is not delayed.

Intermittent squints. There is not the same degree of urgency for these patients since binocular single vision is being maintained for part of the time and so the deviation does not have so adverse an effect on binocular function. If, however, treatment is postponed in these cases, observation should be kept to make sure that the situation does not deteriorate.

Fully accommodative squints. Complete control of the deviation is usually possible by orthoptic treatment alone but this first stage is often best left until the age of approximately five years so that co-operation is better. Binocular single vision is constantly maintained with glasses so that binocular function is not harmed by the delay.

Correction of the deviation

Full binocular function in binocular single vision is most likely to be re-established if these functions have been re-educated and exercised immediately before the visual axes are restored to parallelism. This stage of the treatment should, therefore, follow closely after the orthoptic treatment described above and is achieved by a variety of means.

Surgery. Surgery is inevitably necessary in constant squints and frequently in intermittent squints of a non-accommodative type. As long as there is no suppression and fusion power is strong the patient should be able to control a small residual deviation—true orthophoria being an unlikely result of even the best planned operation—and measures can be taken to assist him.

Prisms. A prismatic correction may be incorporated in the glasses where surgery is not possible (e.g. on general health grounds) or Fresnel prisms (p. 144) may be used as a temporary measure to restore binocular single vision until either surgery or orthoptic excercises render them unnecessary.

Miotics. These are most frequently used for cases of accommodative convergent squint with convergence excess and can also be prescribed for fully accommodative squint. Their action is to induce accommodation peripherally, thus avoiding the central stimulus of convergence.

Orthoptic treatment. One of two lines may be followed according to the type of deviation. In accommodive squint, treatment may be given which exercises accommodation and convergence in varying relationships. In non-accommodative squints the aim of treatment is to teach a voluntary joining of the two diplopic images into one fused impression. The former is an excellent and satisfactory form of treatment but the latter is not widely successful though it can be satisfactory in cases in which the deviation is small.

Consolidating exercises
In the orthoptic department and at home exercises are practised to ensure the steady maintenance of binocular single vision, and in the case of fully accommodative squints this includes training the patient to accommodate without over-converging within the confines of his refractive error.

Observation
It is always good policy during the formative years of childhood to see that no deterioration takes place in the maintenance of binocular single vision.

Cases of uncertain prognosis
The cases for whom no clear prognosis can be formed are those with a congenital or early onset of squint and whose present age is, as yet, too young to allow full investigation. Every opportunity for developing binocular single vision should, however, be given to a patient—and the very fact that he is so young makes that more possible, since the formative years of reflex development are not yet passed.

Visual acuity
Refraction should always be carried out, but refractive errors (apart from gross anisometropia or other unusual errors) are not usually of aetiological significance and it is unlikely that any glasses prescribed will influence the deviation. Any amblyopia must be treated at as early an age as possible in order to enable proper foveal development.

Surgery
These cases should have early operation if there is to be a chance of restoring binocular single vision; this means, preferably, before the age of 2 years.

Observation
Periodic appointments should be made so that cases achieving

binocular single vision can be checked for normal development during childhood and so that any recurrence of amblyopia in cosmetic cases can immediately be halted.

Cases of poor prognosis

Such cases will show one or more of the many factors which prevent the restoration of binocular single vision—though it may well be unwise to place patients in this category before a trial course of treatment has been carried out in an attempt to overcome the barriers to binocular single vision. The management of these cases varies according to age.

Children

Visual acuity. Refraction is an essential part of the management of these cases and glasses may, as well as improving the visual acuity, so reduce the size of the deviation that the cosmetic problem is solved. Regardless of the prognosis for binocular single vision, amblyopia should be treated wherever possible in cases in whom the risk of permanent pathological diplopia does not arise. It is difficult to justify allowing a child to grow up with amblyopia which might render him virtually blind in the event of an accident to the fixing eye later in life.

Orthoptic exploration. A short trial course of orthoptic treatment may be necessary before it is certain that the prognosis is poor, but once that is apparent, there is little point in persevering to improve only slightly binocular function which is bound to remain inadequate.

Surgery. This is indicated if the cosmetic appearance warrants it, for a noticeable squint can lead to great unhappiness, since it has a socially ostracising influence stronger than is found with most other physical deformities. In deciding on the question of surgery, the actual appearance is more important than instrument measurements and the significance of the glasses should also be remembered. It is plainly a mistake to operate in order to gain parallel visual axes without glasses for a child who is highly hypermetropic and will be wearing the glasses, with an unsightly divergence, all day.

Observation. The refractive correction, the cosmetic appearance and the visual acuity should be reviewed during childhood.

Adults

There should first be a careful investigation of adults with longstanding squint and no fusion, for whom surgery is considered for cosmetic reasons, to determine the risk of post-operative diplopia. There may well be a peripheral area of suppression preventing pathological diplopia with the present angle of squint but inadequate suppression to prevent it closer to the fovea. This is particularly true in large deviations with gross amblyopia. The test may be done by cocainising the eye and rotating it into the straight position with forceps or, alternatively, the orthoptist corrects the deviation with prisms while the patient is asked if diplopia occurs. The orthoptist is then able to report to the ophthalmologist if there is a risk of diplopia post-operatively—and, if the exact correction of the squint results in diplopia she may be able, by testing an under-correction with prisms, to predict the degree of residual deviation which would not cause it. In cases of divergent squint, which many ophthalmologists prefer to leave consecutively convergent, a report on the risk of diplopia with the deviation overcorrected would be made.

Persistent post-operative diplopia causes immense distress to some people and none at all to others and, if it is known to be a possibility, the ophthalmologist must decide whether it should be discussed with the patient. Discussion often makes the diplopia more noticeable and it can be argued that the patient would never have 'looked for it' if he had not been warned of the possibility. The other point of view is that the patient should be informed of the possible complications arising from his desire for a purely cosmetic operation.

PARETIC SQUINTS

A considerable number of patients show a paretic element in that they exhibit either an A or a V phenomenon (p. 96). The way in which this influences the management depends on the type of deviation with which it is associated.

Cases of latent deviation which are complicated by an A or V phenomenon may simply show an increase in the latent deviation either on elevation or depression, or the deviation may actually become manifest in that direction. Surgery is inevitable if the phenomenon causes troublesome symptoms.

Intermittent or constant squints with all grades of binocular vision have a good prognosis. The presence of either an A or a V phenomenon must be taken into account when planning surgical treatment to achieve binocular single vision.

In constant squints with no binocular function the problem is purely cosmetic and if the phenomena are not marked they can be ignored.

Paretic squints may most easily be considered depending upon whether the palsy was congenital or acquired.

Congenital paretic squints

These may attend at a very early age or may not seek treatment until later in life, and their management varies accordingly.

Children

Young patients with a congenital paresis causing a constant manifest squint should, on the whole, be considered for treatment on the same prognostic basis as are the cases with concomitant squint. The exceptions are the cases with a compensatory head posture, which will be discussed separately. Management of paretic cases differs from that of non-paretic in certain respects.

Visual acuity and orthoptic treatment. The prescription of glasses is not likely to influence the deviation of paretic origin, and decisions concerning occlusion and orthoptic treatment are based on the same principles as for concomitant squint.

Surgery. This is inevitable if a paretic squint is to be eradicated, and so cases with good prognosis should be operated on in order to achieve binocular single vision. This may well be planned as a series of operative steps because frequently there is both a vertical and a horizontal deviation to be corrected. Cases with poor prognosis may require surgery for cosmetic reasons; if the primary deviation is horizontal it is often considered wise to operate on the horizontal deviation only in the first instance, as any vertical element is frequently reduced to a cosmetically acceptable size by this measure. If the primary deviation is vertical, however, one would undertake vertical surgery first.

Observation. It is necessary to check that the post-operative result is retained and to watch for any recurrence of amblyopia.

Children with a compensatory head posture. An abnormal head posture has been adopted by these patients in order to retain binocular single vision in spite of a paresis of one or more of the extra-ocular muscles. Sometimes the deviation has proved too great for this compensatory mechanism, and both a manifest squint and the head posture are present. These cases should be operated on according to their prognosis or cosmetic indications.

The children who have retained binocular single vision by means of the head posture should almost invariably have ocular surgery so that the compensatory mechanism is no longer necessary and permanent deformities of the spine are prevented. These patients do not usually have amblyopia, but facultative suppression may well have developed in the direction of the manifest deviation and this should be overcome by orthoptic treatment before the operation is carried out.

Adults

Older patients with congenital paretic squints are, again, best considered from the management point of view according to whether or not an abnormal head posture has been adopted.

Those without a compensatory head posture and a manifest squint will have a poor prognosis because of the long neglect of a congenital deviation. Careful tests for the risk of post-operative diplopia should be carried out before advising surgery for cosmetic reasons. The procedure for this has already been described (p. 130).

Adults with a compensatory head posture. Patients for whom a head posture has enabled the normal development of binocular single vision are in quite a different category, but their treatment is not as straightforward as it would have been in childhood because by now the abnormal head posture may have caused secondary neck and spinal changes. Surgery is, therefore, usually advised only if symptoms are being experienced—either ocular ones, due to the difficulty of maintaining binocular single vision, or physical ones, due to the maintenance of the abnormal head posture.

Pre-operative treatment to overcome the suppression, which will be present when looking into the direction of the squint, is necessary for the best results. Surgery may be planned in more than one stage and post-operative treatment to consolidate the maintenance of binocular single vision with the head held straight may be considered desirable. Patients often have difficulty in holding the head straight at first after a life-time of an abnormal posture, and occasionally physiotherapy may be considered to help them to overcome it.

There is a group of adults with a slight congenital vertical muscle palsy who maintain binocular single vision without a compensatory head posture. With advancing years they may suffer symptoms—headaches, eye strain, diplopia. In a few cases surgery may be indicated but more usually a small prismatic correction will relieve symptoms.

Acquired paretic squint

Patients with acquired paretic squint should have a good prognosis for the restoration of binocular single vision provided that there is not a recent neurological basis for the palsy. But, of course, if the onset was during the developmental years and attendance is delayed, management will be based on the cosmetic considerations already described for congenital squints.

Those patients who attend, whether as children or adults, with a recently acquired paretic squint, must be managed in a specialised way.

Observation

Particular reference is made to the cause, and any suggestion of a neurological basis for the palsy must be thoroughly explored. The ocular condition should be recorded periodically if the onset is recent because acquired paretic squints usually make at least some degree of recovery and the surgeon must be confident that no further spontaneous recovery is likely before he plans any surgical intervention. In cases due to orbital injury, for example blow out fractures, there should be no delay in treatment if there is obvious enophthalmos and herniation.

Diplopia

There will be either transient or constant diplopia and this is specially distressing in an adult who may also be unwell and confused. Careful orthoptic assessment can provide some immediate diagnostic clues both after injury and in the early stages of suspected disease or lesion. Repetition of tests will then record progress or regression. It should be possible to establish which muscles or nerves are affected, to differentiate between innervational and mechanical restrictions and also to differentiate between peripheral and neurological disturbance.

While performing ocular movements note should therefore be made of any lagging, impairment or nystagmoid effort on pursuit movement and also of any impairment of saccadic movement or failure of voluntary gaze movements. Disjugate and conjugate movements should also be examined and any disruption of vergences reported. Convergence may be normal in spite of failure to adduct either eye or there may be convergence palsy in spite of good adduction. Accommodation should always be tested and pupil size noted in each eye. These facts together with doll's head phenomenon, optokinetic responses and, if necessary, caloric investigations, complete the clinical picture.

An abnormal head posture. Possibly a position could be found whereby an area of single vision is more conveniently placed, but this is only likely in mild paresis.

Occlusion. This is an alternative and has the advantage of preventing the development of suppression which can occur with the adoption of an abnormal head posture, particularly in the direction in which diplopia remains.

Occlusion of the unaffected eye forces the patient to attempt to use the paretic muscle and this is either an advantage or not depending on the aetiology of the palsy. Fixing with the affected eye does, however, carry the disadvantage of resulting in the proprioceptive disturbance of 'past pointing' in which there is faulty assessment of the position of objects due to the excessive stimulus required to take up fixation.

Occlusion of the affected eye is, therefore, the more comfortable.

Patients are often happier to alternate the occlusion as it encourages them to feel that either eye is still capable of functioning, but where spontaneous recovery is taking place occlusion should not be worn constantly, but regarded as an aid to comfort and safety only.

Fresnel prisms. These can be of considerable value in achieving single vision during the 'waiting period' of medical progress in paretic squint and in cases of restriction due to thyroid dysfunction. The variability of the deviation is a problem but comfort in at least two useful positions (e.g. for reading and television) affords great relief.

Orthoptic investigations. The reports on these visits will provide the best guide to the progress of the case in a series of Hess charts and, where appropriate, in fields of binocular single vision. The orthoptist may also be able to show the patient how to join his diplopia and make use of the gradually enlarging field of binocular single vision, for the importance of reassurance should not be forgotten at this stage; the months of waiting can be long and depressing for the patient.

Treatment

Active intervention only becomes necessary if improvement halts before the spontaneous recovery is complete. A minimum period of six months after the onset of the palsy is usually desirable to ascertain that full spontaneous recovery is not going to take place. In certain cases due to disease this period may have to be considerably longer while the patient has treatment to stabilise the medical or neurological condition. After some head injuries recovery may continue for two years or more and it is advisable to delay surgery until a minimum static period of three months has elapsed after initial improvement, during which regular Hess charts for comparison are important.

Surgery. This is the most desirable form of treatment since it restores, as exactly as is possible, the proper balance of the extra-ocular muscles. In advising operation the surgeon should remember that binocular single vision in all positions of gaze is an ideal he may only achieve after several operations, if at all, and he should perhaps be hesitant to advise surgery if non-alignment remains only in a small and relatively unimportant field of vision. Thus a patient who maintains comfortable binocular single vision on depression and has a manifest deviation on marked elevation only should possibly be congratulated on his good fortune and discharged by all but the most experienced surgeons, since surgery to restore ocular balance in elevation may disturb it in the infinitely more important depressed position. This point arises particularly in children whose parents naturally notice the elevated position more while the child is small.

Prisms. If, for some reason, surgery is contraindicated, prisms may be prescribed. The prismatic correction of paretic squint is not an easy task as there is frequently some inconcomitance and thus prisms which are suitable for one position of gaze are not for another.

Orthoptic treatment. Very little can be gained by orthoptic treatment of paretic squint, although it is possible to show a patient how to move a fixation object away from a position in which fusion occurs to try and enlarge the field of binocular single vision. This probably has more psychological than physical value.

UNILATERAL APHAKIA

Specialised management is required for unilateral aphakia in that the problems arising from the condition are specialised. The cases in question are those who, having one normal eye, are unilaterally aphakic following, usually, traumatic cataract.

The problems

Amblyopia may develop rapidly in young patients because of loss of stimulus to the affected eye.

Loss of binocular function also takes place rapidly and, even in adult cases, is a common characteristic in patients with more than four month's time lag between the development and removal of a traumatic cataract.

Deviation of the affected eye—usually convergent in children and divergent in adults—follows the loss of binocular vision.

Aniseikonia amounting to approximately a one-third enlargement of the aphakic image is optically inevitable. This is far in excess of the 5 per cent difference which can normally be overcome.

The management

Cataract extraction must be performed as soon as possible after its development since the prognosis for the restoration of binocular single vision deteriorates very rapidly indeed if the cataract is of greater than the three months duration.

An orthoptic investigation should be carried out to ascertain whether binocular single vision will be established if contact lenses are prescribed. The patient is fitted with a trial contact lens and routine orthoptic examination will determine if the patient has binocular single vision with the lens or, in cases of manifest squint, whether fusion is still present. For these patients fusion assessment with red and green goggles is as valuable as a major amblyoscope investigation. An alternative method to the use of trial contact lenses is the use of special aniseikonic slides on the major amblyoscope.

The prognosis for the binocular outcome of the case is formed as a result of the orthoptic investigation of fusion.

Selection for contact lens fitting or intra-ocular lens implant as a permanent measure should be made on the basis of the prognosis for binocular single vision. Failure to regain binocular single vision will lead either to constant diplopia or to a deep suppression of the aphakic image and these patients therefore, do not benefit from the fitting of permanent lenses. Both forms of lens correct the visual acuity and the contact lens may be either soft or hard, though the soft variety require extreme care in supervision. Contact lenses have the advantage over intra-ocular lenses in that they are safer and can be removed, whereas the intra-ocular lenses must be decided upon before the cataract surgery and are contra-indicated in younger patients.

Correction of the deviation is not always necessary. The hypertropia which is common in the early stages of the investigation and during the preliminary fitting very usually disappears and small horizontal deviations can be controlled when the final lens is fitted. However if, in the presence of fusion, a manifest deviation persists, surgery will be required to regain binocular single vision.

Perseverance with wearing the lenses is an important facet of success; symptom-free binocular single vision may take several months to achieve and in some cases may be assisted by orthoptic treatment to improve fusional reserve and convergence.

12

Non-surgical treatment of squint

The broad plan of the management of cases of squint has now been described and in this chapter the methods of carrying out the various non-surgical forms of treatment which are available will be considered.

TREATMENT OF BINOCULAR POTENTIAL

This aspect of the treatment of squint is carried out entirely by the orthoptist and therefore only a brief account of the methods used is appropriate here. During the treatment the aim is, of course, to establish steady normal retinal correspondence, strong fusion and good stereopsis (first having eradicated any abnormal binocular tendencies which may be present) so that binocular single vision is a practical possibility when the visual axes are restored to parallelism. Most of the treatment is given on the major amblyoscope, on which bi-foveal stimulation can be achieved in spite of the presence of a manifest squint.

Abnormal retinal correspondence

It is very difficult to eradicate abnormal retinal correspondence but several forms of major amblyoscope treatment have been devised in order to convey to the patient that the superimposition of images received by non-corresponding points is incorrect and to establish gradually a correct correspondence between the foveae. The use of after images and Haidinger's brushes have been turned to this purpose and a major amblyoscope has been adapted to include the mechanisms for creating these entoptic phenomena. Between attendances for the treatment total occlusion must be worn constantly to prevent continued stimulation of non-corresponding points. In some cases with a tendency to abnormal retinal correspondence this may prove successful, but harmonious abnormal retinal correspondence in a cosmetically acceptable squint is certainly better left alone as it is in itself a form of binocular function for which there may be no substitute.

Normal retinal correspondence

This is established by carefully controlled objective treatment on the major amblyoscope. The orthoptist continually stimulates the two foveae with simultaneous perception slides (e.g. the lion and the cage) until the patient is able to demonstrate normal retinal correspondence by correctly adjusting the tubes himself to the exact angle of squint to achieve superimposition.

Suppression

All foveal suppression must be overcome if binocular function is to be efficient and, again, this is done mainly by major amblyoscope exercises. Graded slides are used and the patient manipulates one tube of the instrument himself, 'chasing' the picture which is in the orthoptist's control in order finally to achieve effortless superimposition of the foveal images. This treatment is accompanied by occlusion between appointments in order to prevent the re-suppression which would inevitably occur without it.

Fusion

Exercises for fusion may be given when one is confident that retinal correspondence is normal, but it will only become strong as all suppression is eradicated. On the major amblyoscope slides depicting similar images are fused at the angle of squint and the range over which this can be maintained is gradually increased by exercising binocular convergence and divergence. Similar exercises can be carried out on a variety of stereoscopes and other instruments and the prism bar may also be used. Where small degrees of suppression persist centrally it is important to encourage good peripheral fusion to ensure the maintenance of gross binocular function.

Stereoscopic vision

This may be encouraged on the major amblyoscope and on stereoscopes using slightly dissimilar images.

Pathological diplopia

Patients with the ability to fuse should be taught to recognise pathological diplopia in the presence of a manifest squint for two reasons, firstly to ensure that all the pathological suppression induced by the squint has been overcome and, secondly as a guide to the patient after the deviation has been corrected so that he may be aware of whether he is maintaining binocular single vision or not. Exercises to teach its recognition include stimulation involving the peripheral areas of suppression (in contrast to the earlier exercises involving the foveal suppression). This is done with stimulation on the major amblyoscope by locking the tubes set for orthophoria so that the fovea of one eye and the periphery of the other retina are simultaneously stimulated. Much use is also made of red and green goggles and prisms in homework exercises.

It is highly dangerous to teach a patient to recognise pathological diplopia before determining whether he is capable of fusion—unless he is so young that re-suppression could be expected in the event of failure to establish binocular single vision. Persistent pathological diplopia in the absence of fusion was one of the outcomes of the early enthusiasm for orthoptic treatment before there was a full understanding of the factors influencing prognosis.

The duration

Treatment to re-establish binocular function will of course, vary with the degree to which it had degenerated. In the case of a child with a weak demonstration of normal retinal correspondence three or four weekly treatments will show whether the progress warrants a full course of exercises, and a further six or eight attendances might be expected to restore functions to the point where binocular single vision can be hoped for. However, if fusion is moderately good and suppression not very dense results will be quicker, while a tendency to abnormal retinal correspondence will necessitate a preliminary course of treatment lasting several weeks.

TREATMENT TO RESTORE BINOCULAR SINGLE VISION

If binocular single vision is to be regained by the patient with a squint, treatment must be given in order to render the visual axes parallel so that the potential binocular function may be put to use. It is true to say that in most cases this will be achieved by surgery, and this large subject will be dealt with in the following chapter. However, in certain groups of squint, non-surgical measures can be taken which will enable the control of the deviation and, in effect, convert a manifest squint into a latent one. The essential preliminary to this type of treatment is that the potential binocular function should be strong and therefore treatment to control the deviation should be delayed until the earlier stages are completed.

The accommodation/convergence relationship

For patients with squints of the accommodative type the accommodation/convergence relationship is the most important approach to the nonsurgical adjustment of the visual axes. (It is, of course, totally ineffective in squints of non-accommodative or paretic origin).

It is believed that the relationship between accommodation and convergence is controlled by a convergence mechanism rather than by an accommodative one. In order to maintain clear binocular single vision elasticity of this relationship is essential. A patient with a convergence tendency will find it necessary to inhibit convergence in relation to accommodation (negative relative convergence) while a patient with a tendency to diverge must use it in excess of accommodation (positive relative convergence). Refractive errors also make demands on the elasticity between the two functions.

There is a limit to the amount of negative relative convergence that an individual can exert and, therefore, if the AC/A ratio (p. 3) is high an accommodative squint may result. These patients require to exert an abnormally large amount of convergence in order to achieve a given amount of accommodation. There are various methods of measuring the AC/A ratio (descriptions of which are not within the scope of this book as this falls into the work of the orthoptist) but one may suspect that if the deviation, measured by the prism cover test, is 10^{Δ} greater for near than for distance a high AC/A ratio exists—and the greater the difference in deviation, the higher the AC/A ratio.

The AC/A ratio may be altered temporarily by miotic treatment and more permanently by surgery.

Miotic treatment

In certain cases this method of treatment may influence the AC/A ratio; in other cases surgery may prove to be necessary. Miotics bring about a peripheral accommodative effect, increasing the influence of innervation to the ciliary muscle. In view of the decreased innervation thus required to achieve each unit of accommodation, there is a comparable decrease in the accommodative convergence which is induced, which is to say that there is a lowering of the AC/A ratio (but as the affect of the drug wears off the AC/A ratio returns to its original value). In addition, the miosis which results is possibly beneficial by increasing the depth of focus.

There are two groups of patients for whom miotic treatment is principally used: in accommodative squints with convergence excess, in order to prevent over-convergence for near fixation with glasses (and, possibly, control the deviation without glasses too), and in small residual convergent deviations post-operatively. The ideal pre-requisites are strong fusion and stereopsis, the recognition of pathological diplopia and a deviation no more than moderate in size, but it is worth a short trial of miotic treatment for cases who are too young, as yet, for the ideal preliminary orthoptic treatment. In addition, miotics may be used to help gain control of fully accommodative squints in patients who have difficulty in achieving it by other means.

Pilocarpine. The drug first used in this work was pilocarpine 2 per cent t.i.d. but it is now considered disappointing and is no longer widely advocated except for post-operative treatment.

Phospholine iodide. P.I. 0.06 to 0.25 per cent nocte is more satisfactory and fear of the side-effects is diminishing; the dose is reduced in strength and frequency as binocular single vision is stabilised.

It is desirable to introduce P.I. at the weakest strength increasing to the full dosage after the preliminary effect on accommodation has taken place. The effect will be seen within two weeks if it is going to be successful, but reduction of the strength should not begin for at least a month and then will be continued gradually over the following few months. The patient may be under miotic treatment for six months, the strength of the drug being reduced first and then the frequency.

Orthoptic care, concentrating on convergence and its relationship with accommodation, should be continued for the first few weeks of miotic therapy and supervision continues to be important throughout the reduction period to ensure firm control of the overconvergence.

Surgery
Should miotics be initially unsuccessful or if, after the course of miotic therapy, the deviation recurs, surgical treatment is indicated. The anaesthetist should always be informed of the use of these drugs.

Optical treatment
Adjustments to the spherical correction worn can be used to a certain extent so that the accommodation required is that which is associated with the correct amount of convergence to maintain binocular single vision. This of course can only be done if the visual acuity remains satisfactory.

Fresnel lenses. After the visual acuity and the cover test have been compared with a small range of possible lenses in a trial frame, the correction can be adjusted with Fresnel lenses if it is found that a slightly higher or lower correction than that prescribed results in binocular single vision. These plastic membranes, constructed and used in a comparable manner to Fresnel prisms (p. 144), are available in positive and negative spherical powers and are invaluable. Adjustments of this nature should only be temporary and should be discontinued once binocular single vision has been restored and consolidated. This type of treatment as an isolated measure is satisfactory in some cases of partially accommodative squint, but it is also of great value post-operatively.

A cut crescent of a Fresnel lens creating a bifocal correction may be used to prevent over-convergence on near fixation in cases of accommodative squint with convergence excess, but this is not widely practised in Britain. The cover test is repeated for the near position while gradually increasing the hypermetropic correction and if it is found that a reading correction restores binocular single vision it may be prescribed. This again is viewed as a temporary measure and the reading correction should be reduced as rapidly as possible while retaining binocular single vision. For this reason the lower segment, which should reach the pupil, is affixed to the ordinary lens for easy replacement.

Orthoptic accommodative treatment
The patient may be taught to control a convergent deviation by means of the accommodative convergence mechanism with orthoptic treatment. It can prove successful in cases of small degree convergent squint of the convergence excess type but is mainly used for patients with fully accommodative squint, who can learn to control the deviation without glasses by this method. These patients may have achieved binocular single vision spontaneously with the correction of their hypermetropia but in some cases it may have been as a result of surgery or miotic treatment. The orthoptist teaches the patient to relax accommodation so that there is no inducement to over-converge and, with the pathological diplopia which has been previously taught, the child will know that he is maintaining binocular single vision by virtue of the fact that he sees a single image. At this stage the image is, of course, blurred, and further treatment aimed at teaching the patient to dissociate accommodation and convergence and thus to achieve a clear image will be necessary (see Treatment to Consolidate Binocular Single Vision, page 146).

Prismatic correction of the deviation
The prescription of prisms results in bifoveal stimulation in spite of the presence of a squint, and this can be a useful form of treatment. As well as providing relief from diplopia, it encourages binocular single vision where surgical correction is undesirable or delayed. It is also used as a temporary measure during the treatment to teach fusional control so that the degree of deviation can be lessened in the first instance; the strength of the prisms is then gradually reduced as fusional control improves.

Fresnel prism. This is a convenient plastic membrane, the principle of which is that the continuous surface of a conventional prism is replaced by a series of steps and thus the thickness of the traditional prism is reduced to as little as 1 mm (Fig. 29). They are supplied in small sheets which can easily be cut to fit a spectacle lens. The scope of

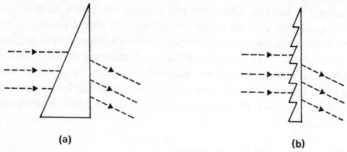

(a)   (b)

Fig. 29 Diagram of (a) a conventional prism and (b) a Fresnel prism

prism correction is thereby considerably widened as the membranes are of negligible weight and cosmetically acceptable even in the highest power (30$^\Delta$). In addition, part of a lens only need be covered where a deviation requires correction in one direction or at one distance. They are simply applied by pressing on to the back of the spectacle lens (under water to prevent the formation of air bubbles) and can be quickly removed or changed. However, they have the disadvantage of reducing the visual acuity, usually by one or two lines of Snellens distance type, and this may be unacceptable.

Fusional control of the deviation

As an isolated procedure this is of very limited value and is confined almost entirely to patients who already maintain binocular single vision in one position—either for near or for distance fixation. These patients, who must recognise pathological diplopia when squinting, can be shown by the orthoptist how to fuse the two images either with the help of the prism bar, which is gradually diminished, or by slowly extending the range over which binocular single vision is maintained, the appearance of pathological diplopia warning the patient if he squints. Instruments such as the Remy separator and stereogram cards are used and success is achieved in selected cases in which the maximum deviation is never very large. It should be stressed that this type of treatment, used in association with treatment based on relative convergence, with prismatic treatment and with surgical procedures, is of very great value indeed.

A combination of several methods

It may be desirable to combine various forms of treatment in order to restore binocular single vision; thus a patient may control a deviation by a combination of miotic therapy and fusional control exercises or by optical means accompanied by orthoptic accommodative treatment and, although the subject of surgery is so important as to warrant a separate chapter in this book for its consideration, it must not be regarded as a separate entity. The most skilful of surgeons must allow that he cannot precisely predict the exact degree of deviation the operation will correct; however, this element of uncertainty gradually reduces with skill and experience until many cases are left with visual axes so near to orthophoria that the patient controls the deviation as a latent one. But, by virtue of the fact that a combination of methods is available, other cases, with slightly larger post-operative deviations, can learn to control the residual squint and maintain binocular single vision.

Post-operative treatment

In those cases to whom binocular single vision is not immediately restored by surgery post-operative treatment is of great value. This treatment is more effective if instituted in the immediately post-operative period and for this reason it is most important to have the orthoptic department in close communication with the hospital ward.

Fresnel lenses adjusting the amount of accommodation required (and thus influencing the convergence) can be used in accommodative cases to increase a hypermetropic correction or reduce a myopic one in post-operative convergence; alternatively to reduce a hypermetropic correction or increase a myopic one in post-operative divergence. This (particularly where a myopic correction is concerned) is only a temporary measure and must be accompanied by orthoptic treatment to consolidate the effect so that the Fresnel adjustment can be reduced and discontinued.

Fresnel prisms will deflect the stimulus to the fovea and can be used in non-accommodative cases, for whom spherical adjustments are valueless. The lowest strength of prism which will result in binocular single vision is worn. The patient must have fusional control exercises in the orthoptic department so that the prisms can be reduced as quickly as possible since their prolonged use is undesirable.

Fusional control exercises may be sufficient without optical aids, when twice-daily orthoptic treatment is desirable in the first few days post-operatively.

Miotics can be of great value in residual accommodative convergent squint and tend to be preferable to the use of Fresnel lenses. This form of treatment can be started immediately post-operatively.

TREATMENT TO CONSOLIDATE BINOCULAR SINGLE VISION

Binocular single vision can be restored to a patient having potential binocular function in a variety of ways but it will often be disappointingly transitory if the achievement of parallel visual axes is not followed up by measures to consolidate the binocular single vision. In addition, this further course of treatment may help the child who is wearing + 3.0 DS or less to discontinue glasses. This stage of treatment consists of improving the fusional reserve, the convergence and the dissociation of accommodation and convergence.

Fusion
Improvement of fusional reserve, both positive and negative, is of importance because it will enable a patient to control without symptoms any remaining latent deviation.

Binocular convergence
It is essential that binocular convergence is maintained to at least 8 cm in order to prevent a secondary convergence insufficiency occurring later in life. Convergence can be improved in several ways: by fusional training, by simple convergence to a near point while watching an object such as a pen and, most important, by exercises which dissociate accommodation and convergence.

Convergence and accommodation
The relationship between accommodation and convergence is of the utmost importance and forms the major part of treatment in many patients who have regained binocular single vision. The importance of this relationship in the maintenance of binocular single vision (p. 3) must never be forgotten and, although this form of treatment is particularly used in those whose squint was accommodative in nature, it also plays its part in divergent deviations.

Relative convergence
This is the ability to adjust the convergence while maintaining a fixed amount of accommodation and is governed by the fusional vergence reflex.

Prisms. While the patient reads a card of near test type, thus maintaining static accommodation, a base-in prism bar will demand reduced convergence (or negative relative convergence) and base-out prisms increased convergence (or positive relative convergence) if binocular single vision is to be maintained.

Lenses. These may be used in a similar way, the convergence remaining static on the near and distant test type while increased accommodation is demanded by concave lenses and reduced accommodation by convex lenses. This used to be regarded as 'relative accommodation' but (since experiments indicate that accommodation is only achieved by an act of convergence) it is now considered that a preliminary alteration of both accommodation and convergence has taken place followed by the 'fixing' of accommodation and then the relative reduction of convergence.

Bar-reading. Since it is very simple to use at home, bar-reading is a much-used orthoptic exercise for this purpose. The 'bar' is held between the page and the face and acts as a control to check that binocular single vision is maintained because, as long as this is the case, physiological diplopia will occur and the bar will not impede reading; if binocular single vision is surrendered, one bar only remains and it will obscure part of the print on the page. In accommodative squints the patient reads gradually reducing print, demanding gradually increasing accommodation if it is to be distinguished. Finally, the use of concave clip-on lenses of increasing strength will exercise accommodation in excess of convergence.

Other instruments. Various devices such as the Holmes and Asher Law stereoscopes, the diploscope and stereogram cards can also be used to exercise positive and negative relative convergence and the wide diversity of techniques which have been evolved illustrate how very important this aspect of orthoptic treatment is.

These exercises of relative convergence may form the largest part of the treatment of fully accommodative squints, gradually resulting in less and less reliance on the hypermetropic correction for clearly defined binocular single vision. Adjustments for up to three dioptres of accommodation can usually be acquired so that patients with low or moderate hypermetropia and a fully accommodative squint can learn to dispense with the glasses or become less dependent on them.

The duration
Treatment to consolidate binocular single vision will vary considerably in length from case to case. Patients with non-accommodative squints may require only three or four attendances while those with accommodation/convergence disturbances may well take over twice as long. The success, as well as the duration of this stage of treatment depends to a large extent on the conscientious use of homework exercises, which are fundamental to progress.

THE ROLE OF THE ORTHOPTIST

Non-surgical treatment is, of course, mainly carried out in the orthoptic department. However, in addition to the technical aspect of conducting the treatment the orthoptist has been trained to be selective and is able to form what is usually a valuable opinion on which particular aspects of the treatment available are best suited to an individual case. Thus the direction of a patient through the possibility of occlusion, pleoptic, orthoptic, optical, miotic and surgical treatment should be the result of close consultation between the ophthalmologist and the orthoptist.

13

Surgical treatment

INDICATIONS FOR SURGERY

There are three main reasons for operating upon squints. The first is to achieve binocular single vision, the second is to relieve symptoms, and the third is for cosmetic purposes. Cases will be considered under the following headings: those with a good prognosis, those with an uncertain prognosis, those with a poor prognosis and those with special problems.

Cases with a good prognosis

These comprise patients in whom binocular function is demonstrable and any amblyopia has been overcome.

Concomitant squints

A *constant squint* should be eliminated by surgery as soon as there is equal visual acuity so that the developing binocular reflexes can be firmly established and anomalous reflexes avoided. Operation should, therefore, be undertaken without delay. Surgery is normally unilateral, involving both the horizontal recti in the originally deviating eye.

Intermittent squints do not give rise to the same urgency, as binocular function will not be so rapidly undermined. In convergent deviations with convergence excess, surgery is undertaken only after miotics and orthoptic treatment have either been proved inadequate, or are judged to be unsuitable. Those with divergence weakness will require surgery. Divergent squints normally require surgery, the timing of which gives rise to controversy; while some advocate delaying surgery until the patient is old enough fully to co-operate with pre- and post-operative orthoptic treatment, others consider that the intermittent deviation should be eradicated as early as possible. No body of opinion would support delaying surgery if the binocular function showed signs of deteriorating.

In contrast to surgery for constant squints, operation on these cases is usually bilateral; the lateral recti being adjusted if the deviation occurs in the distance and the medial recti if it occurs for near.

Inconcomitant squints

Congenital paretic squint. Cases with congenital palsy which have a good prognosis are normally characterised by a compensatory head posture. Such cases may first attend either in childhood or as adults. Children should have surgery both in order to render the head posture unnecessary and to prevent decompensation in later life. Adults only require surgery if symptoms are being experienced.

Surgical treatment may well be planned in stages and the usual procedure is firstly to weaken the overacting contralateral synergist to the affected muscle, secondly to weaken the direct antagonist and possibly to strengthen the affected muscle itself.

The prognosis for binocular single vision in all directions of gaze is particularly good in these cases if treated in childhood. Adults may have difficulty in abandoning the postural habits of a lifetime.

Acquired paretic squint. Cases of paretic squint due to a recent lesion of the nerve supplying the extrinsic ocular muscle have potentially a good prognosis because, if the lesion has occurred after the full establishment of binocular vision, restoring the visual axes to parallelism will effect, in many cases, a reasonable binocular result. No surgical interference, however, should be undertaken until (a) the cause of the paresis is known, (b) time has been allowed for the maximum recovery to be achieved, and (c) a full orthoptic investigation has been completed with the essential diagnosis of the affected muscle or muscles. It would obviously be inapproprate to operate upon a paretic squint caused by a neurological disease such as disseminated sclerosis, a cerebral condition due to aneurysm or neoplasm or any other condition which may produce a transient or a progressive paresis.

The following are the cases of acquired ocular paresis which are suitable for surgical treatment if full spontaneous recovery does not take place and the deviation has remained static for six months.

1. Those due to fractures of the skull which involve the oculo-motor nerves.
2. Those due to local injury to the orbits, where the ocular muscles are involved in fractures or displacements of the orbital walls. The orbital injury itself should always have immediate treatment. Also occasionally those due to trauma caused by surgery to the frontal sinus or the surgical treatment of detachment of the retina.
3. Those due to inflammatory conditions of the brain and meninges

which have resolved but left a residual ocular palsy, as in tuberculous meningitis and encephalitis.

4. Those due to vascular disease such as cerebral aneurysm, as in ophthalmoplegic migraine and cerebral haemorrhage or thrombosis in patients with arteriosclerosis.

5. Those due to involvement of the muscles themselves, as in exophthalmic ophthalmoplegia when the endocrine dysfunction has been stabilised.

In cases of acquired ocular paresis there is an overaction of the contralateral synergist and, with the passage of time, there is a contracture of the direct antagonist of the paralysed muscle and defective action of the contralateral antagonist. It will be found that the operation indicated will be a weakening of the action of the contralateral synergist or of the contracted ipsolateral antagonist. In addition, the action of the paresed muscle or of the defective contralateral antagonist may be strengthened. The operation may have to be carried out in stages before a satisfactory result is achieved.

There will always, however, be some cases with contra-indications to surgical treatment, especially among the elderly, where the general condition may be poor; relief of symptoms by prisms or by occlusion may be the only available measure.

The object of the operation should be to restore parallelism of the visual axes in the primary position. It must be remembered that full restoration of movement in all directions of gaze cannot always be achieved, but an important aspect is the increase of the field of binocular single vision: particularly in the most important directions—usually straight ahead and depression.

Cases with uncertain prognosis

These are the cases which are too young to enable binocular function to be demonstrated clinically or else are so young that an early operation to restore the visual axes to parallelism might enable binocular single vision to develop.

Concomitant squint

If a squint is present constantly in the infant and is associated with a bilateral habitual weakness of the lateral recti and a tripartite field of fixation, operation may be required early to enable the possible development of binocular single vision. Such cases should be watched carefully over the period from 6 to 18 months, as often improvement takes place after alternating occlusion for a very brief period (p. 108). Operation is indicated if the situation is static. The other advantages of early operation in these cases are firstly that there is an immediate improvement in the child's appearance; secondly, there is less psychological trauma to the child at this age and, thirdly, the motor changes secondary to longstanding convergence are avoided. The disadvantage is that if binocular single vision does not develop, too liberal surgery may result in divergence later.

In the older age group it is recognised that the earlier the onset of the squint and the longer the delay in treatment the worse is the prognosis. Therefore the advantage of immediate operation is obvious, since the period of squinting is reduced, binocular vision has a chance to develop and it may be possible to complete the treatment before school age, which is economically sound and psychologically advantageous.

Inconcomitant squints

The congenital paretic squint without compensation presents as a paresis of one or more of the extrinsic ocular muscles. The deviation may be simply a vertical squint or combined with a horizontal deviation. They present no signs of binocular vision, that is, there is no compensatory head tilt or turn, and binocular function is difficult to demonstrate clinically because of the inconcomitance. Once the visual acuity is equal it is important that these cases should be operated upon early to restore the visual axes to parallelism in all directions of gaze. If this is done it is possible for some cases to develop binocular single vision.

It is often difficult to ascertain which muscle or muscles are primarily at fault, but in planning surgery it should be remembered that an entirely satisfactory result will not be achieved unless the primary vertical deviation is corrected. Surgery will possibly have to be carried out in several stages.

Cases with poor prognosis

These are cases in which there is some permanent barrier to the development of binocular single vision. Examples may be found in those with intractable amblyopia, with no evidence of fusion, or with defects in the visual pathways, i.e. obstacles to vision in the media, corneal opacities, lens opacities, macula lesions, optic atrophy, etc. In such cases surgery is only indicated if the cosmetic appearance warrants it.

Concomitant squints

In the constant concomitant squint where operation is required for cosmetic reasons the operation for the convergent type should be designed to straighten the axis of the defective eye. This is usually done by weakening the action of the medial rectus and strengthening the action of the lateral rectus. Care should be taken to avoid fully correcting or over-correcting the deviations as such cases may tend to diverge with the passage of time.

If the convergent squint in a young child with high hypermetropia is operated upon, less adjustment is necessary as such cases tend to diverge consecutively with the passage of time, whereas the longstanding squint which has developed contractures may require a larger operative correction.

The small angles of esotropia where there is a tendency to anomalous correspondence may require operation to adjust the visual axes accurately. In a few cases normal retinal correspondence may develop, but on the other hand the results are often disappointing, the eyes often returning to the original deviation and so, if the cosmetic appearance is good, operation may be contraindicated. Some useful form of binocular vision with abnormal retinal correspondence or peripheral fusion may develop without operation.

In divergent squints the adjustment of the visual axis in the deviating eye can be more liberal as, without fusion, the eyes will tend to resume again the divergent position.

Inconcomitant squints

In these cases there is often a marked vertical deviation as well as a horizontal one. It is important for the cosmetic appearance to adjust the vertical deviation as accurately as possible. It is often found that the vertical element in these cases is, in itself, a barrier to fusion and occasionally, by adjusting this and removing the barrier, some degree of binocular function may develop.

In certain cases of traumatic paretic squint occuring in adult life fusion has been lost and it may be more satisfactory to leave a deviation post-operatively which separates the diplopia into the blind-spot area—though very precise full corrective surgery has been known to aid fusion recovery.

Special cases

Alternating sursumduction

This is a condition in which, on dissociation, the embarrassed eye deviates progressively upwards, but reverts to its original position when the dissociation ceases; it is also known as dissociated vertical divergence. It may be found with a manifest vertical deviation, a latent or manifest horizontal deviation and, frequently, with latent nystagmus. The aetiology is obscure. In the management of these cases the alternating sursumduction is often ignored and treatment is considered for the associated deviation; however, the faden operation of Cüppers is meanwhile gaining popularity; this involves suturing the superior rectus to the sclera 14mm behind is insertion, thus reducing its power of rotation.

A and V phenomena

It would seem that these phenomena (p. 96) spring from a variety of causes and, before planning surgical treatment, some assessment of the possible aetiology should be made. Surgery should, therefore, only follow an exhaustive investigation of the ocular movements. The operative procedure selected will also depend on the experiences and preferences of the individual surgeon. However, it is of value to outline some of the recommendations to be considered.

Gross examples are often associated with imbalance of the oblique muscles and, in that case, surgery on them is indicated and is often successful. There is a belief that the phenomena are due to a primary weakness of the vertically acting muscles which particularly affects their secondary horizontal actions; abnormal insertions or incorrect alignment of oblique muscles may also produce a torsional element.

Surgery to weaken the over-acting obliques is recommended with adjustments to the insertions if necessary to correct the plane of action. In examples of the phenomena showing a relatively small variation in size on elevation and depression (15° or less) it may be sufficient to raise or lower the lateral or medial recti insertions in the course of horizontal surgery. Thus in a V phenomenon with esotropia, the insertions of the medial recti would be lowered when carrying out the bilateral medial rectus recession.

Duane's retraction syndrome

This congenital condition is the outcome of fibrosis of the extrinsic ocular muscles or of their fascial connections, which prevents full and free movement of the globe. Its true aetiology may not, however, be simply musculo-fascial since investigations show co-contraction of extraocular muscles caused by paradoxical innervation, which could be the result of a supranuclear lesion. The signs vary in individual cases and three types can be recognised, but the salient characteristics are limited abduction and adduction with a retraction of the globe on attempted adduction, accompanied by narrowing of the palpebral fissure. In some cases it is compensated for by an abnormal head posture.

The result of surgical intervention is so disappointing that it is usually only undertaken if the condition is symptom-producing, or if the abnormal head posture is unsightly. Some improvement of the position of a convergent eye may be achieved by temporal displacement of the insertions of the superior and inferior rectus muscles combined with a recession of the medial rectus of the affected eye.

The superior oblique tendon sheath syndrome (Brown's)

These cases are characterised by a gross or total lack of elevation on adduction coupled with a remarkably small—or even no—hypotropia of the affected eye. This eye also shows a downdrift on adduction, and in some cases there is also an updrift of the unaffected eye in its abducted position. Diagnosis may be confirmed by a forced duction test under general anaesthesia when it is found that the affected eye cannot be elevated from the adducted position.

The defect is caused by an anomaly of the sheath surrounding the superior oblique tendon; it may be short, fixed to the trochlea, thickened at the posterior end, or blemished by a nodule, and any of these abnormalities can mechanically prevent the globe from rotating freely into the elevated position on adduction.

Surgical treatment is designed to weaken the superior oblique muscle, usually by a free tenotomy of the tendon or, in slight cases, a division of the sheath but results are often disappointing and minor degrees are better left alone.

Alternate day squint

This rare condition (also known as cyclic or circadian squint) has, usually, a 48-hour cycle of variation between a 'straight' day with normal binocular single vision and a 'squinting' day with a marked manifest deviation, when little or no fusion or stereopsis are demonstrable, but there is no diplopia. Refractive error is usually insignificant and the deviation may become constant after some months if not treated. Surgery on the maximum angle has proved successful.

Nystagmus

In conditions of manifest nystagmus, the adoption of a certain head position may limit the excursion of the nystagmus. It has been found that by adjusting the muscles in each eye so that the visual axes correspond to the primary position with the head straight, the appearance can be greatly improved. For example, if the nystagmus becomes almost stationary when the head is turned to the right, i.e. with the eyes in a position of laevo-version, the right medial and the left lateral recti are recessed; in addition, a resection of the right lateral rectus and the left medial rectus may be required in marked cases.

Latent nystagmus only occurs when the eyes are dissociated and is occasionally found in cases of convergent squint and is frequently associated with alterating sursumduction. By correcting the deviation in the primary position, the nystagmus often diminishes.

Nystagmus blocking syndrome. The nystagmus blocking (or compensation) syndrome occurs in some cases of congenital manifest nystagmus as a means of minimising the condition. The fixing eye is adducted, with a resultant head turn, within the first few months of life, and the hypertonacity of the medial recti results in esotropia of the other eye with all the usual characteristics of manifest squint plus a bilateral pseudo-palsy of abduction. Response to a medial rectus recession and lateral rectus resection of the non-fixing eye may be satisfactory.

Unilateral aphakia

After the removal of a cataract, there is a tendency for the aphakic eye to diverge. Where efforts are made by means of a contact or intra-ocular lens to restore binocular single vision in a young adult following a traumatic cataract, surgical adjustment may be required to restore parallelism to the visual axes. In such an event, the soft or the microcorneal contact lens is considered more satisfactory than the haptic lens since refitting is unnecessary with them, whereas, due to conjunctival scarring, the fitting of a haptic lens might have to be changed post-operatively.

Ptosis

Drooping of the upper lid is usually due to underaction of the levator muscle and may be associated with weakness of the adjacent superior rectus. Cosmetic and postural considerations will influence surgery. If the pupil is covered, binocular function will be affected and amblyopia may be found.

Pseudo-ptosis. This is apparent in an eye which is hypotropic and disappears when the unaffected eye is occluded so that the hypotropic eye assumes the primary position to take up fixation. It also occurs to a minor degree in Duane's retraction syndrome and occasionally the close proximity of the upper lid to the pupil of a hypertropic eye may give the same appearance. No surgical interference to the upper lid is indicated in any case of pseudo-ptosis.

SURGICAL PROCEDURES

It is outside the scope of an orthoptic handbook to describe in detail this vast subject. It is one which can only be learnt from specialised writings, practical guidance and personal experience. However, a brief résumé will be made of the various operations designed to weaken or strengthen the action of the extra-ocular muscles.

Weakening operations

Recession. This is an operation in which the muscle is detached from the globe at the insertion and replaced further back.

It is quite the commonest form of weakening operation to be carried out on the horizontal and vertical rectus muscles. A recession has a very marked effect on the superior and inferior recti, so that comparatively large vertical deviations can be eliminated by a suprisingly small adjustment. It is also true to say that recessing a medial rectus has a greater effect than recessing a lateral rectus.

This operation is gaining favour as a controlled procedure for weakening the inferior oblique in contrast to the myectomy.

Tenotomy. This is an operation in which the tendon is cut. Quite its most valuable use is to weaken the superior oblique, but it may also be employed on the lateral rectus in cases of marked divergent squint. It is never used on the medial rectus except in cases of strabismus fixus. Another form of the operation is to carry out a partial tenotomy, or to guard the effect of a complete one by a loose retaining suture.

Myectomy. This is an operation in which a portion of the muscle length is removed; it can be performed to weaken the inferior oblique.

Marginal myotomy. This is a procedure in which incisions are made in the margins of the muscle concerned. It is possible to use this cautious technique on the horizontal or vertical rectus muscles but it is now rarely advocated as its results are unpredictable.

Strengthening operations

Resection. This is an operation in which the muscle is detached from the globe so that a portion may be removed before the muscle is reattached to its original insertion. This is a highly successful strengthening operation and quite the most commonly performed; it can be used on all the muscles.

Advancement. This is an operation in which the muscle is detached from the globe and a new insertion is made further forward. It has no advantage over resection as a primary operation (although it may be combined with a resection to heighten the effect in gross deviations) but it is of value as a second procedure for a muscle on which an overliberal recession has been performed.

Tucking. This operation consists of folding a portion of the muscle or tendon upon itself and securing the fold with mattress sutures. It is not advocated for the rectus muscles and, even for the obliques, it is now rarely used.

Transplantation. This operation is only considered for complete paralysis of the lateral rectus. The procedure is that strips are taken from the medial third of the superior and inferior recti, detached from their insertion, passed under the outer two-thirds of the muscle and stitched onto the upper and lower margins of the lateral rectus insertion, so that the strip is made taut. The latter muscle is also resected.

PRINCIPLES OF SURGERY

When planning the surgical procedures to be followed for a case of squint, it should be remembered that there is a variety of circumstances which influence the effect of a given operation, so that no hard and fast ratio of millimetres of recession or resection to degree of deviation adjusted can be drawn up. Care must be taken in recessions not to reattach the muscle behind the equator and the resection should not cover more than 8 mm. The result of overliberal surgery may be a consecutive deviation and limitation of movement of the operated eye. The operation should, therefore, be planned with careful reference to the full clinical picture and not merely to the size of the angle of the squint.

The principal factors to be borne in mind are:

Unilateral squint is usually treated by unilateral operation unless the angle of squint is so large that it would demand gross surgery on the muscles of one eye; in these circumstances, it would be better to divide the operative procedures between the two eyes.

Alternating squint of moderate degree is considered best treated by bilateral, symmetrical surgery, but if the deviation is large, surgical adjustment of one eye, probably followed by a similar procedure on the other eye, is desirable.

Inconcomitant squints may warrant unilateral surgery, in spite of alternation, the first measures being taken on the eye which shows the larger deviation when the other eye is fixing.

Convergent squints without binocular function which are operated on for cosmetic reasons, should be left residually convergent compatible with good appearance. This is because of the natural tendency to diverge which might ultimately result in an unsightly consecutive divergence, should the deviation be fully corrected in childhood. Cases with binocular function should, of course, have surgery planned with a view to eliminating the deviation so that binocular single vision may be taken up post-operatively.

Accommodative squints should be considered with special reference to the necessity of the glasses from the visual point of view. If they are being worn primarily to reduce a squint and would not have been required in other circumstances, surgery for the squint and release from glasses should be advised. The operation will, of course, be planned for the deviation without glasses.

Constant divergent squints without binocular function will tend to re-diverge with the passage of time and therefore surgery should be designed to 'overcorrect' the deviation in the first instance so that a good cosmetic appearance is retained throughout life. As was remarked for convergent squint, if a binocular, rather than a cosmetic result is hoped for, the aim of operation will be to eliminate any deviation and no calculation to 'overcorrect' the angle should be made.

Intermittent divergent squints should not be regarded as requiring more tentative surgery than a constant deviation and the operation should be planned on the basis of the maximum deviation elicited by prisms and, if necessary, the dissociating effect of a temporary occlusion. In cases of the divergence excess type with a high AC/A ratio (which is common) bilateral lateral rectus recessions are preferable to a unilateral recession and resection.

In paretic squint, if binocular single vision in all directions of gaze is an unlikely outcome, surgery should be planned to ensure binocular single vision in the most important position (usually depression) and leave any residual diplopia in the least important position (usually elevation).

Secondary vertical squints frequently are eradicated by the surgery on the primary horizontal deviation, so that vertical surgery is best not undertaken in these cases until this assumption has been proved incorrect. This will not, of course, be true if the vertical deviation is primary.

A younger patient shows a greater post-operative effect from a given operation than does an older one.

High hypermetropia tends to increase the effect of surgery.

The size of the deviation influences the effect of surgery, large deviations being corrected with relatively less surgery than small ones.

Simultaneous surgery, that is, a recession and resection carried out in the same session, will have a greater combined effect than if the two operations are performed with an interval between them.

Further surgery may be planned after approximately one week if the earlier operation has proved to be inadequate and the deviation remains undercorrected. However, there is a risk involved if further surgery for an apparent overcorrection is carried out with the same speed, as a gradual reduction of the immediate result is possible and the final effect of an operation is not certain until one or two months later.

These pointers will serve to indicate the very personal and individual problem which each case of squint presents to the surgeon and to explain the variation in techniques advocated by different ophthalmologists. Operating on a squint is not the simple, rule-of-thumb procedure it was all too frequently considered to be not many years ago, and the successful treatment of patients suffering from a disturbance of binocular single vision may only be achieved by the careful and painstaking co-operation of ophthalmologist and orthoptist throughout whatever optical, orthoptic and surgical treatment the case may demand.

Index